Joachim Hasse

Surgical Treatment of Bronchial Carcinoma

Screening Methods, Early and Late Results

With 23 Figures and 46 Tables

Springer-Verlag
Berlin Heidelberg New York Tokyo

Priv.-Doz. Dr. med. Joachim Hasse
Kantonsspital Basel
Departement Chirurgie
Klinik für Herz- und Thoraxchirurgie
Spitalstrasse 21
4031 Basel, Switzerland

ISBN-13: 978-3-642-70979-1 e-ISBN-13: 978-3-642-70977-7
DOI: 10.1007/978-3-642-70977-7

Typesetting, Printing and bookbinding: Graphischer Betrieb Konrad Triltsch, Würzburg
2124/3140-543210

Foreword

If a consecutive series of patients with lung cancer is followed up until the decision is made about therapy, it emerges that the role of surgery is quite small. Only a very limited proportion will ultimately qualify for rationally conceived surgical therapy; most patients are inoperable. In a series of 397 patients investigated at our hospital, 78% were inoperable on the basis of preoperative evaluation and a further 3% proved nonresectable at thoracotomy; therefore, only 19% were suitable for resection.

On the other hand, surgery is still thought to offer the best, if not the only realistic chance of cure. The question "operable or not?" is therefore of vital importance for the individual patient. The answer to this crucial question must be based on valid guidelines for patient selection and preoperative evaluation, and it should be clearly defined what extent of resection is necessary in order to realize any curative intention.

In 1972 a thorough analysis of the literature revealed that resection of bronchial carcinoma – although 40 years old – was being undertaken with very variable indications. There was hardly any systematic staging, and assessment of results was hampered by the fact that most communications in the literature were based on retrospective analysis.

It was therefore that Dr. Hasse has conceived a prospective study on the surgical therapy of bronchial carcinoma at our hospital. The protocol was established with the aim of defining the efficiency of surgery, based on a standardized investigational program with standardized guidelines for indication and surgical principles concerning technique and extent of resection. It also outlined a program of prolonged postoperative surveillance and follow-up in order to assess late results. The report on the results of this prospective study forms part of this book.

Dr. Hasse has shown that good results can be achieved following the guidelines established in this protocol. Operative mortality has been low, although surgical indication has been generous with respect to reduced functional reserves, advanced age, and other preoperative risk factors as long as the criteria for curative resection are fulfilled. Accurate preoperative assessment of these risk factors, expert anesthesia, and adequate postoperative treatment of high-risk patients, applying knowledge and experience gained in part from cardiac surgery, contributed greatly to these favorable results.

This book represents a very important contribution to a better understanding of a controversial problem and offers helpful information to all physicians and surgeons engaged in the surgical treatment of bronchial carcinoma.

Basel, February 1986

E. Grädel

Preface

Surgery remains the treatment of choice for bronchial carcinoma, and indeed bronchial carcinoma represents the predominant indication in the whole field of noncardiac thoracic surgery. Numerous publications have been dedicated to this topic; however, this volume covers new ground. Usually, single aspects of the diagnosis and treatment of bronchial carcinoma are addressed by experts on particular problems, but we have intended to draw a more complex picture of a clinical series which, by virtue of its limited size, allowed us to review the various problems arising in clinical reality, starting with the task of correct staging, interpretation of histologic descriptions, and characterization of surgical procedures. With the wealth of information collected by continuous documentation, we also became attracted by the idea of discussing a variety of common or episodic complications and their attempted or successful resolution. We do not claim to have been exhaustive in every instance; we preferred to consider as many as possible of the questions arising in the course of our daily work, rather than concentrating on details. Finally, it seemed worthwhile not only to present survival figures, but also to examine the circumstances of early and late death and to analyze the patterns of failure.

I am gratefully indebted to Professor E. Grädel, head of the Cardiac and Thoracic Clinic at the University of Basel and my teacher in cardiac and thoracic surgery. In the early 1970s, he provided the stimulus for a prospective investigation with the aim of establishing or confirming generally valid principles in the selection for and practice of operative treatment of bronchial carcinoma. The result of this fundamental proposition was the setting up of a standardized diagnostic program which was then adopted by all physicians and surgeons involved in preoperative care.

I also wish to express my sincere gratitude to Professor B. Spiessl, head of the Oral Surgery Clinic at the University of Basel, the principal editor of the German edition of the TNM rules (UICC) and initiator and principal editor of the TNM Atlas. As one of the pioneers in tumor classification in many discussions concerning the crucial necessity of documentation and the use of unambiguous definitions, he encouraged me to publish these data and my thoughts about further improvements.

I would like to thank my friend Dipl. Ing. Chem. J. Slanicka for his advice and generous help in regard to the statistical workup and for the practical execution of the statistical analyses. Likewise, Mr. G. Rechsteiner deserves my thanks for his excellent graphic work. Finally, I should like to thank the staff of Springer-Verlag for the preparation and generous illustration of this monograph.

Basel, February 1986 Joachim Hasse

Table of Contents

Introduction

There is a vast body of literature dealing with the surgical treatment of carcinoma of the lung. Varying opinions have been expressed on a range of specific problems relating to diagnosis and patient selection, and there has been even greater diversity in the results that have been reported. Evaluation is made especially difficult by the fact that almost all studies to date have been retrospective and therefore omit certain information that is pertinent to the characterization of patient groups [178].

This problem is illustrated by a 1976 study of Stanford et al. [327], which reports a 5-year survival rate of 48.8%, and a 1974 study by Weiss [355] indicating a survival rate of 22%. Neither study gives information on the selection and prevalence of the different tumor stages. One study emphasizes the positive results of surgical treatment, while the other expresses skepticism as to its value. Without more information on the circumstances which led to these results, the data obtained from large operative series are not meaningful.

For some time there have been international attempts to standardize the histologic classification and staging of tumors as a prerequisite to the comparison of therapies. Although Nohl [241] showed as early as 1960 that treatment outcomes in lung cancer correlate with the extent of the tumor and the occurrence of regional metastasis, even many recent publications make no reference to the question of tumor staging. Where staging is considered, it is very often been based on modifications of the accepted international TNM system.

It is our intent in the present study to avoid these disadvantages. Our study is prospective in character, and the diagnostic program, rules for patient selection, and operative principles are standardized. Some minor changes in diagnostic procedures were implemented during the almost seven years of patient enrollment in the study, but we do not feel that they compromise the homogeneity of the series. The changes were necessary responses to clinical discoveries or newly available examination methods.

We have devoted considerable space to the issue of tumor staging and the practical implementation of the staging system. In addition, we have attempted to clarify the ambiguous definitions that necessarily occur in such a system by introducing our own interpretations.

We are privileged to be able to present this study in the form of a monograph. This enables us to explore many details and aspects that usually have to be omitted in a study of this kind. Besides presenting results that are of purely statistical interest, we are able to address a number of specific problems based on evaluations of individual case reports.

A key element in the study is the strict follow-up program that was maintained for a minimum of 6 years and a maximum of 13 years after surgery. Thus, we are dealing with true-response data with regard to five-year survival rates in surgically treated lung cancer patients.

Chapter 1

General Characteristics of the Operative Series

Patients

From the beginning of 1972 to the end of September, 1978 (publication of the Third Edition of the TNM Classification of the WHO, introducing stage IV disease [340]), 206 consecutive patients with preoperatively or postoperatively confirmed primary carcinoma of the lung were treated surgically at the Clinic for Cardiothoracic Surgery of the University of Basel, Switzerland. While only 17 operations were performed in 1972 (the year in which the clinic expanded its services to include both cardiac and noncardiac thoracic surgery), the rate in subsequent years rose to 30 or more carcinoma operations performed annually.

The male patients in our series predominated over the females by nearly 10:1 (187 to 19). The average patient age was 59.5 years, with a range from 32 to 75 years. The under-50 group accounted for only 13.5% of the total population. Nineteen patients were over 70 years of age. Almost half the patients were between 60 to 69 years of age (Fig. 1).

The present study is comparable to many others in its scope. The 10-year report of the Geneva University Clinic covers 253 operations with 204 resections [216], with an average patient age of 60.3 years. In a Bonn University Clinic study spanning more than 20 years, the annual rate of operations is 30, and the average patient age is 58 [103]. The collaborative study of 16 German surgical hospitals, consisting of 12 university hospitals and 4 specialty clinics, covers 1164 resections in the 5-year period from 1970 through 1974. The average resection rate per institution and year in that series was 15 [20]. The 10-year re-

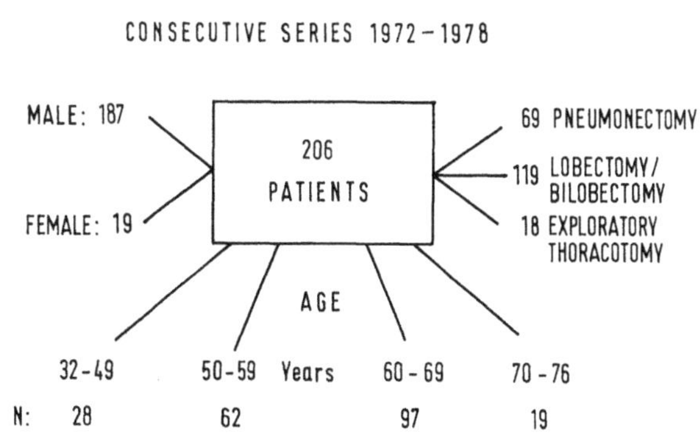

Fig. 1. Age and sex distribution of the patient population, and the number and types of procedures performed

port of Kirsh et al. (1976) from Ann Arbor, Michigan, covers 437 patients [173]. Thus, the yearly operating rate is somewhat higher but is still comparable to that in our study. The same applies to the 7-year report of Massachusetts General Hospital, Boston, which covers 322 patients [363]:

Number and Types of Operations

A total of 212 operations were performed on 206 patients, 6 of whom required secondary resections during the period of entry or later in the follow-up period. In 18 cases the resection was abandoned because the cancer was judged to be technically inoperable when the chest was opened. This corresponds to an 8.7% overall incidence of purely exploratory thoracotomies. But as the graph in Fig. 2 shows, the percentage of exploratory operations declined from approximately 30% to about 6% as the study progressed. The introduction of mediastinoscopy (see p. 38) obviously was instrumental in that trend.

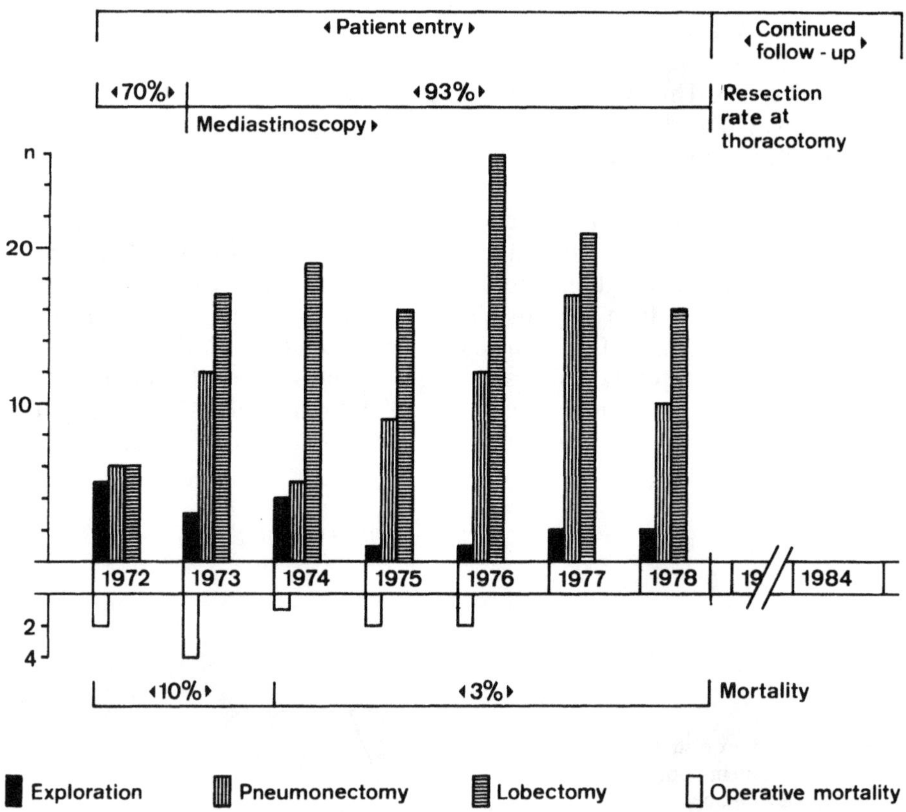

Fig. 2. Yearly rate of operations, frequency of exploratory thoracotomies, and mortality

Pneumonectomies

Sixty-nine patients (36.7%) underwent a pneumonectomy as their primary operation. In addition, three secondary, complementary pneumonectomies were performed: for recurrence of the carcinoma in two patients, and for double carcinoma in one patient. Three patients underwent previous operations for malignant (2) or benign (1) disorders on the ipsilateral side.

Partial Resections

This category includes lobectomies, bilobectomies of the right lung, and one wedge resection (which hereafter is counted among the lobectomies for purposes of discussion and statistical evaluation). Ten of the bilobectomies involved the upper and middle lobes (upper bilobectomy), and six involved the lower and middle lobes (lower bilobectomy). Three patients who underwent primary lobectomies later had to have a lobectomy on the contralateral side because of further malignant disease.

Among the 119 primary partial resections that were performed there were 2 patients who had had previous resective surgery abroad – one lobectomy for neoplasia and one segmental resection for tuberculosis.

A detailed survey of all resections is presented in Table 1.

Table 1

			Primary		Total
Pneumonectomies,			69		
	left	41			
	right	28			
	secondary (complementary)			3	72
Partial resections					
Lobectomies,			118		
	left upper lobe	36			
	right upper lobe	27			
	left lower lobe	16			
	right lower lobe	17			
	right middle	6			
	bilobectomies				
	upper (UL + ML)	10			
	lower (ML + LL)	6			
Wedge resection			1		
	secondary (opposite side)			3	122
Resections			188		194
Explorations			18		18
Total			206		212

Table 2. Preoperative symptoms and their duration

	Less than 3 months	3 to 6 months	Longer	Total
None				54
Cough (new or +)	30	30	17	77
Expectoration (new or +)	26	22	6	54
Hemoptysis	30	13	9	52
Weight loss	36	20	18	74
Chest pain	27	10	2	39
Paraneoplastic syndrome (Fig. 3)	11	3	3	17
Cumulative total	160	98	55	

Symptoms (Table 2)

Fifty-four patients were asymptomatic at the time of the first abnormal chest radiograph. Forty-five of these patients were still asymptomatic at operation, while the remaining nine developed symptoms during observation and/or nonspecific therapy.

Cough (new or worsening), expectoration (new or worsening), and hemoptysis were the most frequent *respiratory symptoms,* affecting between 52 and 77 patients. The most precise time data were furnished with regard to the onset of hemoptysis. Of 52 patients who complained of blood-streaked sputum, 21 stated that the symptom had been present for 3 months or longer. Two patients said they had experienced occasional hemoptysis more than one year before their operation.

The preoperative duration of worsening cough or expectoration had passed the six-month limit in approximately one-third of patients.

The most common *systemic symptom* was weight loss. Significant weight loss was present in 74 patients. In half of cases weight loss was appreciable only in the last three months prior to operation. Only nine patients complained of anorexia.

Thirty-nine patients complained of chest pain. In most cases the chest pain did not correlate with recognizable pleural involvement or tumor invasion on X-rays.

Eighteen patients had complaints referrable to paraneoplastic syndrome (PNS) (Fig. 3). In 17 this was confirmed retrospectively by the postoperative improvement or disappearance of symptoms and objective regression of changes.

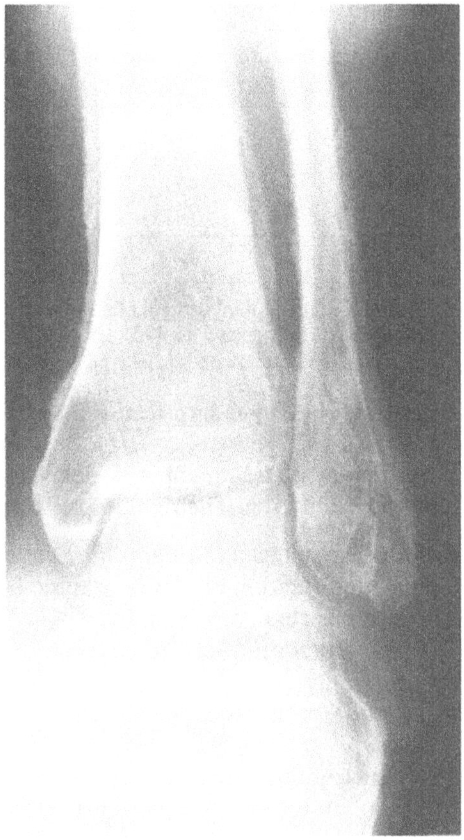

Fig. 3. Example of osteoarthropathy with periosteal calcification. The patient (R. M.) was a 56-year-old man with paraneoplastic syndrome associated with a $pT_3N_0M_0$ large cell undifferentiated carcinoma of the lung (palliative bilobectomy and chest wall resection)

Delay Times (Table 3)

The "delay times" are the intervals that elapsed between the onset of symptoms or first abnormal radiograph and the institution of operative treatment.

In the 54 asymptomatic patients, the detection of abnormalities on photofluorograms or other "routine" chest radiographs (insurance examinations, preoperative films, postinjury films, checkups) marked the start of the delay interval. Ten patients were referred promptly for further evaluation and surgery within one month. In 26 cases the delay time was 1–3 months, and in 18 cases it was longer.

In 52 patients the delay was iatrogenic. These were cases in which obvious radiographic abnormalities were documented prior to the onset of symptoms. Surgery was delayed for 1–3 months in 20 patients, up to 6 months in 12 patients, up to 1 year in 9 patients, and longer than 1 year in 11 patients.

Table 3. Delays in surgical treatment

	< 1 month	1–3 months	Up to 6 months	Up to 12 months	> 12 months	Total
A	10	26	8	7	3	54
B		20	12	9	11	52
C		45	11	1	–	57
D		25	8	7	3	43
						206

A: Asymptomatic patients, incidental radiologic finding
B: Symptomatic patients who had seen physician within 2 weeks (iatrogenic delay)
C: Symptomatic patients who delayed seeing physician after onset of symptoms (compound delay)
D: Delay caused entirely by patient, treatment initiated within 4 weeks after presentation

In four cases treatment was delayed when the patients refused further diagnostic evaluation. The remaining delays were based on:

1) failure to detect a radiographic abnormality suspicious for carcinoma;
2) misinterpretation of a radiographic finding as an inflammatory or other noncancerous change;
3) misinterpretation of hemoptysis (e.g., as gingival bleeding in denture wearers);
4) negative bronchoscopies (usually outpatient) performed under local anesthesia;
5) absence of other evidence of carcinoma;
6) trial of antibiotic therapy or expectant observation;
7) lack of communication between different parties involved in the diagnosis;
8) inefficient evaluation protocol.

An analysis of these causes is given in Table 4.

Examples of Delayed Surgical Treatment

a) Prolonged Diagnostic Evaluation

A 48-year-old man (M. E.) presented to his physician with hemoptysis. Chest radiography showed a large density in the right paramediastinal region. The patient was referred for bronchoscopy (hospital A). This was done 2 weeks later as an outpatient procedure and revealed a tumor at the inlet of the middle lobe. Eleven days later the patient was admitted to hospital B, and mediastinoscopy was performed 14 days after admission. The patient was transferred for surgery 2 days later. Supplementary examinations and preliminary treatment took 6 days. Total delay time from presentation to operation: 3 months. The tumor was identified as a stage III squamous cell carcinoma. Patient died 2 years after pneumonectomy from local recurrence and metastases.

b) Misinterpretation of Radiographic Findings

A density was discovered incidentally in the right lower lung of a 66-year-old woman (A. M.). Tomograms were interpreted as showing a benign lesion, possibly a tumerculoma, vascular malformation, or small pulmonary embolism. The next chest films were taken 2 years and 9 months later when the patient presented with cough, weight loss, and anorexia. Adenocarcinoma was diagnosed. Five months after lobectomy the patient died from abdominal metastases.

Table 4. Reasons for delay in surgery

Inefficient examination procedure	55
Observation of incidental findings (combined in some cases with communication failures)	30
Misinterpretation of radiographic findings (cf. Fig. 15)	
Unspecified	19
Pneumonia	13
Tuberculosis (with appropriate history)	6
Lesion overlooked	3
Failure to confirm tumor after investigation by	
Bronchoscopy	6
Cytology/biopsy	3
Misinterpretation of symptoms (no evaluation)	
Hemoptysis	4
Other	1
Uncertainty regarding use of radiotherapy or chemotherapy	2
Uncooperative patient	4
Disease and preliminary therapy (surgery, trauma, myocardial infarction, preliminary radiotherapy)	7
	153

c) Prolonged Observation[1]

A 59-year-old man (R. K.) presented with a density in the upper right paramediastinal region. A second radiograph 5 months later demonstrated enlargement of the lesion. Four weeks later, outpatient bronchoscopy with cytologic examination of washings was negative. Another chest film was taken 6 weeks later, at which time the patient was referred for hospitalization with a tumor in the anterior segmental bronchus of the upper lobe, a poorly differentiated squamous cell carcinoma. Delay time from incidental detection to operation: 9 months. Patient died from pneumonia about 4 years later.

d) Combined Causes (Communication/Misinterpretation of Hemoptysis/Prolonged Evaluation)

A faint, 2 × 3-cm density over the left hilus was discovered incidentally on the routine chest film of a 61-year-old man. Further evaluation was recommended, but this recommendation was not properly communicated. Eighteen months later the patient presented to his doctor with hemoptysis. Eight weeks' inhalation therapy was of no benefit. Patient was referred to a specialist, and radiographs showed atelectasis of the left upper lobe. A one-week course of antibiotics did not improve radiographic findings. Patient was referred for bronchoscopy, which showed obstruction of the upper lobar bronchus by tumor. Two weeks later the patient was referred for assessment of operability. Surgery, performed 21 months after the first suspicious radiograph, uncovered an inoperable squamous cell carcinoma. Patient survived another 6 months on radiation therapy.

e) Failure to Confirm Tumor

Photofluorographic screening in a 46-year-old man (F. M.) revealed a density in the right hilar area. Bronchoscopy 6 weeks later showed stenosis of the upper lobar bronchus; biopsy was negative. Repeat bronchoscopy 2 weeks later showed a decrease in the stenosis. Four months later the patient was hospitalized because of marked enlargement of the density. Surgery 6 months after the suspicious photofluorogram revealed an inoperable small cell carcinoma. The patient survived another 6 months on radiotherapy and chemotherapy.

---

[1] See also p. 64–66

Following a careful review of the literature and an analysis of their own observations, Wilde et al. [360] conclude that, in cases where data are available, the delay time from the first abnormal chest radiograph to definitive surgical treatment averages between 4 and 12 months. Similar figures are reported by Gall [90] and by Toepfer and Riedel [336]. The factors which thwart early detection and surgery of lung cancer are detailed above.

Boucot et al. [33] and Weiss and Boucot [354] argue that early detection has little bearing on the long-term result of resective surgery. Indeed, there are patients who have survived long periods after their cancer resection even when surgery was greatly delayed. It would be wrong, however, to take this as proof that early detection and surgery are of no benefit. It must be considered that long delay times tend to select patients whose carcinomas have a low proliferative tendency and a low metastatic potential.

A number of publications on the relatively favorable results of resections of coin lesions that are fortituitously diagnosed, and thus are peripherally located in most instances, further support the value of early detection and intervention [28, 62, 106, 131, 132, 149, 311, 348]. Studies by Ermisch [72], Favez [76], Oeser [246], and Trefny [337] show a correlation between early detection and increased resectability rates.

The importance of early detection is supported on a prospective basis by the Mayo Screening Project [82, 257], the results of which appear to conflict with those of the Philadelphia Lung Project, on which Weiss and Boucot [354] base their conclusions. First it is demonstrated that patients whose lung carcinoma was detected on entry into the study (86 out of 9300) were equally divided between stage I and stage II and had a 3-year survival rate of 65% after resection. Moreover, the mortality rate per 1000 in closely followed patients declined as the study progressed in comparison with controls. Early detection does not appear to improve survival in patients with small cell carcinoma, whose prognosis remains grave. Early detection in itself, then, does not necessarily prolong life [69].

Preexisting and Coexisting Diseases

As one would expect from their high average age, a number of the patients had associated chronic diseases that were already known and treated before their lung cancer was diagnosed. These diseases were known from the patients' histories and were clinically confirmed. Here we shall mention only those conditions that might be presumed to increase the risk of surgical resection. Afterward we shall look at preexisting malignant diseases.

Preexisting Chronic Diseases

This group comprised 80 patients with a total of 97 diseases that appeared to be significant. Pulmonary and cardiovascular disorders were the most common, occurring in 44 and 40 cases, respectively. Preexisting pulmonary disorders

Table 5. Preexisting diseases confirmed by history and clinical findings

a) *Pulmonary*			
Tuberculosis		21	
Under observation, inactive	18		
Active	2		
Treated by segmentectomy	1		
Chronic asthmatic bronchitis		20	
Chronic therapy	10		
Periodic therapy	7		
Silicoanthracosis under observ.	3		
Bronchiectasis (1 segmentectomy, 1 bilobectomy)		2	
Spontaneous pneumothorax		1	
Total			44
b) *Cardiovascular*			
Coronary artery disease		26	
Previous myocardial infarction	10		
Chronic angina pectoris	16		
Atrial fibrillation of unknown etiology		1	
Valvular disease with insufficiency		2	
Significant hypertension		6	
Peripheral arterial occlusive disease		5	
Above-knee amputation for gangrene of toes	1		
Total			40
c) *Miscellaneous*			
Surgically treated head injury		1	
Hemiplegia after hemangioma surgery		1	
Hemiplegia after cerebral insult		1	
Hepatopathy (alcoholic, viral)		2	
Gastritis, duodenal ulcer		2	
Diabetes requiring treatment		4	
Nephrotic syndrome		1	
Thalassemia		1	
Total			13
Total overall:			97

were led by tuberculosis and chronic obstructive disease. The leading cardiovascular disease was coronary artery sclerosis.

More detailed information is given in Table 5.

Malignant Diseases

Fifteen of the 206 patients had one or more malignant diseases prior to diagnosis and treatment of their lung cancer. Five of the patients had previous lung carcinomas, and it was unclear whether the present carcinoma was new or recurrent. If the interval had been short, a recurrence was presumed. These patients are discussed later in more detail.

Table 6. Preexisting malignant diseases

a) Lung carcinomas		
Histology	Treatment	Interval
Squamous	Resection + radiation	1 year
Squamous	Resection, incomplete	2 months
Squamous	Resection	3 years
Adeno	Resection + radiation	15 years
Adeno	Resection	11 years
Total		5

b) Extrapulmonary tumors		
Type/organ	Treatment	Interval
Larynx	Resection + radiation	22 years
Larynx	Radiation	4 years
Larynx	Resection + radiation	2 years
Hodgkin's disease	Radiation + chemotherapy	9 years
Hodgkin's disease	Radiation + chemotherapy	19 years
Cervical cancer [a]	Radium implant	5 years
Cervical cancer	Resection	7 years
Uterus	Resection	8 years
Pancreas	Resection	3 years
Kidney	Resection	7 years
Basal cell carcinoma [a]	Resection	1 year
Total		11

[a] Malignant diseases in the same patient

There also were nine patients who had been previously treated for other types of tumor. Three had carcinomas of the larynx.

The specific locations of the tumors, their modes of treatment, and the delay times prior to surgery are presented in Table 6.

Chapter 2

Oncologic Characteristics

Histology

Basic Types of Primary Lung Carcinoma

Primary malignant tumors of the lung exhibit a variety of histologic characteristics, reflecting the normal cellular makeup of pulmonary tissue. Most of these tumors arise from epithelial and glandular structures of the bronchial and bronchioloalveolar surfaces.

As early as 1924, Marchesani (quoted in Kreyberg [177]) recognized four types of carcinoma:

1) basal cell cancers (corresponding to small cell undifferentiated carcinomas),
2) polymorphocellular cancers (large cell undifferentiated carcinomas),
3) keratinizing squamous cell cancers, and
4) columnar cell adenocarcinomas.

Today this system still forms the framework for the histologic classification of lung cancers. However, continuing observation and histologic examination of lung tumors and refinements of examination techniques have led to the discovery of various cell types that are difficult to fit into the classic scheme. The result is the formation of numerous subgroups which characterize the current generally accepted classification systems of the WHO (World Health Organization, Geneva), WP-L (Working Party for Therapy of Lung Cancer), and NCI (National Cancer Institute Contract Group Lung Cancer Classification, 1977 Pathology Committee) (Table 7a).

These classification systems are contemporary with the period of patient enrollment in our study. The classification system presently used (WHO, Geneva 1981, Supplement [316a]) is shown in Table 7b for comparison.

Distribution of Histologic Types in the Patient Population

The cancer cell types in our series identified by the histologic examination of surgical specimens are listed in Table 8. The nomenclature for these tumors basically follows the scheme of the WP-L. It will be noted that the large groups of squamous cell carcinomas and adenocarcinomas are subdivided according to

Table 7a. Comparison of the histologic classifications of carcinoma of the lung

WHO	WP-L	NCI
I. Epidermoid carcinoma	10. Epidermoid carcinoma	I. Squamous carcinoma
	11. Well differentiated	A. Well differentiated
	12. Moderately differentiated	B. Moderately differentiated
	13. Poorly differentiated	C. Poorly differentiated
II. Small cell carcinoma	20. Small cell carcinoma	II. Small cell carcinoma
1. Fusiform	21. Lymphocyte-like	A. Lymphocyte-like/small (oat) cell
2. Polygonal	22. Intermediate cell	B. Intermediate
3. Lymphocyte-like		
4. Others		
III. Adenocarcinoma	30. Adenocarcinoma	III. Adenocarcinoma
1. Bronchogenic	31. Well differentiated	A. Well differentiated
a. Acinar	32. Moderately differentiated	B. Moderately differentiated
b. Papillary	33. Poorly differentiated	C. Poorly differentiated
2. Bronchioloalveolar	34. Bronchiolopapillary	D. Bronchiolar/alveolar
IV. Large cell carcinoma	40. Large cell carcinoma	IV. Poorly differentiated carcinoma
1. Solid tumor with mucin	41. With stratification	
2. Solid tumor without mucin	42. Giant cell	V. Large cell undifferentiated
3. Giant cell	43. With mucin formation	A. Giant cell
4. Clear cell	44. Clear cell	

Table 7b

1. Squamous cell carcinoma (epidermoid carcinoma) Variant: a. Spindle cell (squamous) carcinoma 2. Small cell carcinoma a. Oat cell carcinoma b. Intermediate cell type c. Combined oat cell carcinoma 3. Adenocarcinoma a. Acinar adenocarcinoma b. Papillary adenocarcinoma c. Bronchiolo-alveolar carcinoma d. Solid carcinoma with mucus formation	4. Large cell carcinoma Variants: a. Giant cell carcinoma b. Clear cell carcinoma 5. Adenosquamous carcinoma 6. Carcinoid tumour 7. Bronchial gland carcinomas a. Adenoid cystic carcinoma b. Mucoepidermoid carcinoma c. Others 8. Others

The World Health Organization Histological Typing of Lung Tumours, Second Edition, Geneva, Switzerland. Published: Am. J. Clin. Path. 77, 123 (1982)

Table 8. Histologic classification (n = 206 patients)

1.	Squamous cell carcinoma		132[a, b]
1.1.	Highly differentiated	4	
1.2.	Moderately differentiated	73	
1.3.	Poorly differentiated	53	
1.4.	With adenomatous elements	2	
2.	Small cell undifferentiated carcinoma		14
3.	Adenocarcinoma		40
3.1.	Highly differentiated	4	
3.2.	Moderately differentiated	16	
3.3.	Poorly differentiated	9	
3.4.	Bronchioloalveolar	7	
3.5.	With scirrhosis	4	
4.	Large cell carcinoma		15[b]
5.	Other and unclassified types		5[b]
Total			206[a]

[a] Histologic findings in 6 patients with multiple or recurrent carcinoma revealed identical types (5 squamous cell carcinomas and 1 adenocarcinoma) and here are counted only once.
[b] Only 131 cases with squamous cell carcinoma are counted for statistical analysis; one patient was lost. Groups 4 and 5 are combined to form the group "Other"

their degree of differentiation. Two squamous cell carcinomas with adenomatous elements are classified among the squamous cell carcinomas, although they probably belong to the rare category of "adenosquamous carcinoma" (category V) of the WHO system. The few tumors that did not fit into any of the four main categories are counted among the large cell undifferentiated carcinomas for purposes of statistical analysis.

Comparing the prevalence of specific histologic types with the operative series of Hinson et al. [135] in England and Matthews and Gordon [211] in the United States, we find that our own data occupy an intermediate position for

Table 9. Prevalence of carcinoma types in different operative series

	Hinson et al. [135]	Matthews and Gordon [211]	Basle series
No. of patients	740	244	206
Squamous cell carcinoma	70.9%	56%	63.1%
Small cell carcinoma	11.6%	3%	6.8%
Adenocarcinoma	8.6%	28%	19.4%
Large cell carcinoma	7.2%	10%	7.3%
Adenosquamous carcinoma	0.7%	2%	1.0%
Other	1.0%	1%	2.4%
Total	100%	100%	100%

most cancers (Table 9). There is a considerable discrepancy in the prevalences of squamous cell carcinomas and adenocarcinomas in the different series, although the total prevalence of both entities is similar, at 80%, 84% and 83.5%, from one series to the next. The prevalence of adenocarcinomas in our series is closer to that in the U.S. study than in the British study. It is uncertain whether this relates to racial and geographic factors or to the difficulty (discussed later) of classifying undifferentiated tumors.

The range of 3% to 12% in the prevalence of small cell carcinoma is probably based on differences in patient selection. In this regard it is interesting to note that the reported incidence of this cancer in autopsy series, 25%–40%, is considerably higher than its prevalence in operative series.

Comparison of Preoperative and Postoperative Tumor Histologies

The foregoing distribution of tumor histologies in our lung cancer patients is based on the examination of resected specimens or, in cases of exploratory thoracotomy, the examination of a specimen obtained by wide excisional biopsy. When we compare these findings with preoperative findings obtained during primary evaluation, we find that the diagnosis or suspected diagnosis made from biopsy or cytology had to be revised in 23 out of 140 cases (Table 10). It is particularly noteworthy that five tumors identified preoperatively as small cell carcinomas had to be reclassified after surgery. This illustrates the pitfalls of the histologic typing of lung carcinomas. Abeloff et al. [1] found that 5 out of 40 patients autopsied at Johns Hopkins Hospital between 7 months and 3 years after initial diagnosis of SCC had 3 squamous cell carcinomas, 1 poorly differentiated adenocarcinoma, and 1 large cell undifferentiated carcinoma in the region of the primary lesion. In four of these patients a small cell carcinoma of the intermediate type had been presumed. Recently Churg et al. [52] reported on 5 additional cases in which electron microscopy showed definite evidence of a squamous cell carcinoma in patients whose primary diagnosis had been small cell anaplastic carcinoma.

Table 10. Revision of histologic diagnoses (23 cases)

Preoperative	Postoperative
Sarcoma	
Large cell undiff.	Adenocarcinoma
Adenocarcinoma	Adenosquamous carcinoma
Small cell undiff.	Squamous cell carcinoma
Unspecified carcinoma	Malignant teratoma
Squamous cell carcinoma	Large cell undiff. carcinoma
Undifferentiated carcinoma	Squamous cell carcinoma
Papilloma	
	Mucoepidermoid carcinoma
Carcinoid tumor	

Table 11. Preoperatively unconfirmed carcinomas

Squamous cell carcinomas:	28 of 132 = 21.2%
Adenocarcinomas:	20 of 40 = 50%
Small cell carcinomas:	9 of 14 = 64.3%
Large cell and other carcinomas:	9 of 20 = 45%

The overall accuracy rate in the diagnosis of cell types in our series is approximately 84% and is comparable to rates stated in the literature [200, 258].

In 66 patients, or about one-third of our total population, the diagnosis of carcinoma remained unproved until surgery or else was limited to the cytologic detection of cells *suspicious* for carcinoma. As we see in Table 11, the percentage of squamous cell carcinomas that escaped histologic detection was relatively small, while half or more of the remaining types were not confirmed until operation. This seemingly high percentage of preoperatively unproved carcinomas does not reflect deficiencies of methodology, but rather is based on the favorable selection of an operative series in which a large proportion of the tumors were still in an early stage. In addition, the peripheral location of the adenocarcinomas and large cell carcinomas accounts for the relatively low success rate of bronchoscopic biopsies and fine-needle aspirations in the diagnosis of these lesions. In the case of small cell carcinoma, the low preoperative yield is not surprising in view of the restrictive patient selection and the tendency for the bronchial mucosa to remain intact in the early stage. Without the shedding of malignant cells, sputum samples will be negative, and endoscopic biopsy is unlikely to be rewarding.

Finally, it is our position that clinical and radiographic evidence of a probable malignant tumor are adequate justification for early operative intervention. We do not feel that a more extensive work-up is necessary in cases of this type.[2]

Problems of Histologic Classification

Although it is proper for the clinician to accept the pathology report with its concluding designation of tumor cell type, he should nevertheless be aware of the difficulties that can arise in the histologic classification of carcinomas. This is particularly true in cases where the pathologic diagnosis can critically affect patient management, as in small cell carcinoma, and when it is necessary to make an analytic evaluation of a treatment modality such as surgical resection.

Recent studies by Spencer [322], Matthews and Gordon [211], Sobin [316], and Lukeman et al. [200] confirm that *well differentiated* squamous cell carcinomas and adenocarcinomas can be diagnosed with a high degree of confidence from histologic sections. The classification of *undifferentiated* tumors is often difficult, however. Large discrepancies in the reported prevalence of specific cell types in clinical and autopsy series support the view that histologic evaluations necessarily involve an element of subjectivity. To quote from Feinstein et al. [77], "The human observer is the least standardized of all the sources of data analyzed in medicine." Many carcinomas of the lung are markedly nonhomogeneous in structure and contain elements which vary greatly in their level of differentiation. The features of the more highly differentiated elements are of greatest diagnostic importance [217]. If well differentiated cells are not found in the presence of marked anaplasia, it may not be possible to distinguish undifferentiated adenocarcinomas or squamous cell carcinomas from a large cell carcinoma by light microscopy alone [200].

It follows, then, that identifying the histologic type of a carcinoma from biopsy or cytologic material can be even more problematic than when the total specimen is available.

Lukeman et al. [200] report that cell-specific diagnoses made on that basis have been accurate in up to 80% of their patients, while in 20% the preoperative diagnosis did not agree with the final diagnosis established by examination of the resected lesion. Very similar percentages are reported by Fischnaller [80] and by Erozan and Frost [73].

Another source of uncertainty is the adenocarcinoma, including the bronchioloalveolar variant. Despite their high degree of differentiation, these tumors are apt to be mistaken for solitary metastases from a tumor of the kidney, thyroid, pancreas, colon, or ovary [211, 322, 367].

The small cell carcinoma, too, is susceptible to diagnostic uncertainty. The characteristic feature of this cancer is its very low degree of differentiation, which is matched by its extremely malignant biologic behavior, i.e., its striking propensity for local invasion and early lymphatic and hematogenous spread. These features explain why small cell cancer has generally come to be regarded

[2] In more recent years, after the completion of this study, the diagnostic yield is considerably higher due to frequent use of transbronchial brush biopsies

as an inoperable disease. It must be understood, however, that even squamous cell carcinomas and adenocarcinomas may contain poorly differentiated cell masses that correspond to small cell carcinoma [52]. Also, it can sometimes be difficult to distinguish carcinoid tumor from small cell carcinoma based on the analysis of small biopsy samples [121]. Lukeman et al. [200] note further that "crush" artifacts caused by the use of small biopsy forceps can mimic the appearance of a small cell carcinoma. Sometimes the electronic microscopy of small cell carcinoma will demonstrate the amyloid that is characteristic of carcinoid-type adenoma [322]. According to Spencer [322], a relationship indeed exists between carcinoids of the lung and small cell carcinoma, which, however, seem to occupy very different positions on the malignancy scale.

Clinical experience confirms that some small cell lung cancers do not take the rapidly progressive course that is expected [322]. Most of these tumors, apparently, correspond to the intermediate type of small cell carcinoma in the WP-L classification although this has not been confirmed by others [48b]. Matthews and Gordon [211] describe its histologic features as follows: The nuclei are larger and less uniform than in oat cell cancers and have small nucleoles. Some cells show marked cytoplasmic structures, and multinucleated giant cells are occasionally seen. Some intermediate-type tumors exhibit foci of large cell carcinoma or other transitional forms with squamous cell carcinoma, while others show rosette formation or tubular structures reminiscent of adenocarcinoma.

We point out these problems in the histopathology of lung cancer to make it clear that the clinician should not base his therapeutic decisions entirely on the literal wording of a biopsy or cytology report. When Salzer [285] published his study on bronchogenic carcinoma 19 years ago subtitled "Fiasco of Histologic Classification", clinicians and even pathologists were far less aware of the problems that exist than they are today. Since then, pathologists have made extensive efforts to establish uniform criteria for the recognition and classification of lung cancers [148]. Even so, the problem of pleomorphism still exists in many bronchogenic cancers [199], and this must be taken into consideration when clinical decisions are made.

Hermanek and Gall [128a] state very emphatically that the diagnosis of small cell anaplastic carcinoma should not be made from biopsy or cytologic material unless confidence is extremely high, so that surgical resection will not be withheld from patients who are potentially operable. At the same time, these authors state that the designation of "small cell" should be applied liberally to *surgical* specimens in doubtful cases so that the potential benefits of adjuvant chemotherapy will not be missed. In other words, attention should be given to clinical therapeutic implications in cases where the histologic classification of a tumor is uncertain.

Tumor Staging

The therapy and prognosis of a malignant disease are determined in large measure by the anatomic extent, or "stage," of the disease at the time of its detection [47, 230, 242]. With carcinoma of the lung, assessment of the *clinical* stage of the disease is based largely on indirect examination methods, and so the reliability of the assessment is limited. Staging in such cases tends to be biased in a favorable direction, because regional spread to the lymphatics and hematogenous metastasis may be present but occult. Studies in surgical populations have the advantage of being able to confirm or exclude lymphatic spread, the earliest form of metastasis in most cancers, through careful, systematic exploration and histologic examination of lymph node specimens. Even in surgical series, of course, uncertainty remains with regard to occult distant metastases.

Besides the identification of tumor cell type, the accurate staging of disease is a necessary preliminary to evaluating our own results and comparing them with other forms of therapy or with other operative series.

Although the TNM staging system of the UICC (Union Internationale Contre le Cancer) has gained wide acceptance and has replaced earlier classifications, it has certain deficiencies that cannot be overlooked and are not easily remedied.

Analogous to the difficulties that exist in the histologic classification of lung carcinomas, the problems of tumor staging are made apparent by the many different classification systems that have been devised.

The TNM principles used by us follow the concepts of the UICC and the AJCCS (American Joint Committee on Cancer Staging and End Results Reporting). This system, which was valid during the period of our study, groups the various T (local tumor extent), N (lymph node involvement), and M (distant metastases) categories into three stages, I through III. The latest version of the TNM system, adopted in Geneva in 1978 and published in the Third Edition of the UICC TNM Classification of Malignant Tumors (Geneva 1978), introduces a fourth stage that is used to designate all cases in which distant metastases (M1) are present. However, the most recent version of the TNM rules of the AJCCS [48a] retains the traditional three-stage classification.

The inclusion of a fourth stage is not new in itself. Ungeheuer and Hartel [342], in a 1968 German-language modification of a 1951 proposal by Salzer, used the designation T4 to denote tumor invasion of extrapulmonic organs. A four-stage classification was also recommended by Goldberg et al. [96] in 1970. Salzer himself continues to use this classification in a study published in 1980 [286]. The German Joint Study on the Results of the Radiotherapy of Bronchial Carcinoma [124] uses the designation T4 with reference to the UICC rules. In an inaugural dissertation by Hauck [122] a fifth category, T5, is used (for pleural effusion with malignant cells), and two numbers are added to designate nodal metastases. Krause [176] uses four designations, N0 through N3, to characterize nodal involvement. In the same year the German Society for Surgery officially recommended that current UICC rules be adopted [64].

Applied Staging Criteria

To preserve the prospective character of our study, we have chosen to maintain the older TNM classification. In cases where it was felt that traditional definitions might allow for multiple interpretations, we added appropriate supplementary comments. We also added subscripts to certain designations, though this does not alter the basic classification:

T 1 Tumor 3 cm or less in diameter surrounded by intact visceral pleura and confined to a lobar bronchus.

T 2 Tumor more than 3 cm in diameter, or any tumor that invades the visceral pleura or extends beyond a lobar bronchus and is at least 2 cm distal to the carina. Any associated pneumonitis or atelectasis must involve less than an entire lung.
Our addition: Tumor 3 cm or less in diameter that extends across the fissure from one lobe to the adjacent lobe (Fig. 4).

T 3 Tumor of any size that extends to an adjacent structure such as the chest wall, the diaphragm, or the mediastinum, or a tumor shown bronchoscopically to be located less than 2 cm distal to the carina, or a tumor associated with pneumonitis or atelectasis of an entire lung or pleural effusion.
Our addition: Tumor located less than 2 cm distal to the carina according to operative findings or pathohistologic examination.

The following subscripts are used to provide a more accurate characterization of T 3 lesions:

a) $T\,3_{mbr}$ Invasion of main bronchus less than 2 cm distal to the carina
b) $T\,3_{pc}$ Pericardial invasion
c) $T\,3_{v}$ Central vascular invasion
d) $T\,3_{th}$ Chest wall invasion
e) $T\,3_{m}$ Other mediastinal invasion

The categories TIS, T 0, and TX are omitted because they are not pertinent to this study or to the majority of surgical investigations.

N 0 No metastasis to lymph nodes
N 1 Metastasis to lymph nodes (Fig. 5):
- $N\,1_{a}$ Intralobar/intersegmental lymph nodes
- $N\,1_{b}$ Interlobar lymph nodes
- $N\,1_{c}$ Hilar lymph nodes

N 2 Metastasis to mediastinal lymph nodes (Fig. 5)
- $N\,2_{tb}$ Superior and inferior tracheobronchial lymph nodes
- $N\,2_{m}$ Other mediastinal lymph nodes

M 0 No evidence of distant metastasis
M 1 Distant metastasis present
- $M\,1_{pul}$ Pulmonary hematogenous metastasis
- $M\,1_{lym}$ Distant metastasis to lymph nodes of contralateral hilus or to extrathoracic nodes
- $M\,1_{h}$ Other hematogenous metastasis

Stage Grouping

Stage I: T 1, N 0, M 0
T 2, N 0, M 0
T 1, N 1, M 0 (not represented in our series)

Stage II: T 2, N 1, M 0
Stage III: Any T 3, any N 2, any M 1

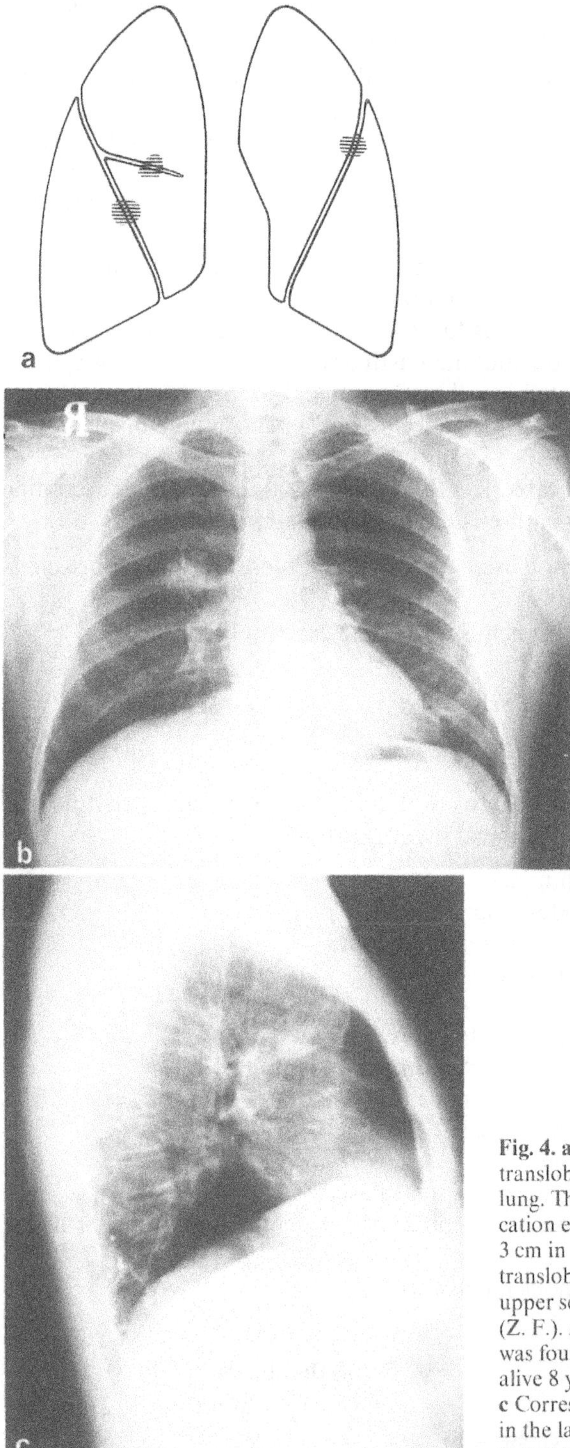

Fig. 4. a Schematic drawing illustrating translobar tumors of the right and left lung. These lesions warrant a T_2 classification even if the carcinoma is less than 3 cm in diameter. **b** Radiograph of a translobar carcinoma of the anterior right upper segment in a 48-year-old man (Z. F.). A pT_2 invasion of the middle lobe was found at operation. The patient is alive 8 years after upper bilobectomy. **c** Corresponding lateral radiograph. Even in the lateral projection, extension of the tumor to the middle lobe is not apparent

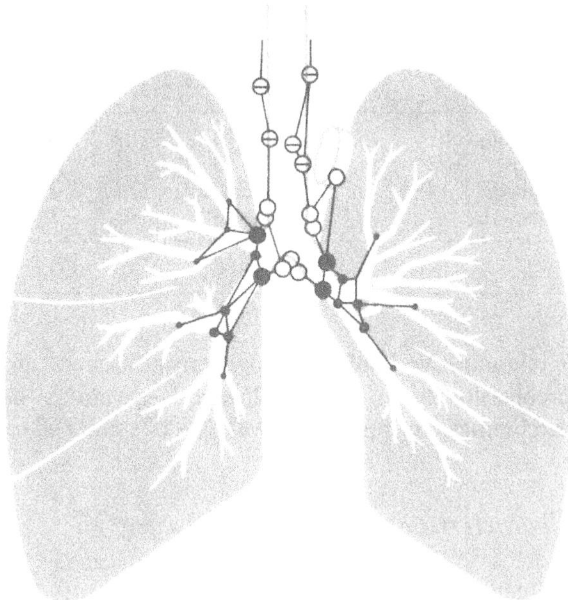

Fig. 5. Map of the pulmonary and regional lymph nodes. • Intersegmental lymph nodes (intralobar lymph nodes) with metastatic involvement: N_{1a}; ● interlobar lymph nodes (with involvement: N_{1b}); ⬤ hilar lymph nodes (with involvement: N_{1c}); ○ tracheobronchial lymph nodes, upper and lower; subaortic lymph nodes (with ipsilateral involvement: N_{2tb}); ⊖ paratracheal lymph nodes (with ipsilateral involvement: N_{2mi})

Table 12. Revised staging of patients according to operative findings (cf. Henney et al. [127])

	Stage I	Stage II	Stage III
Preoperative	186	–	20
Postoperative	91	43	72

Staging Results in this Series

Preoperative and Postoperative Classification (Table 12)

At the conclusion of the preoperative evaluation, 186 of the 206 patients were diagnosed as having stage I cancers. However, intraoperative findings and histologic examination of surgical specimens indicated a more advanced tumor stage in 95 of these patients. In 43 of the patients, involvement of intralobar or interlobar lymph nodes (N 1) warranted a classification of stage II disease. Fifty-two patients were identified as having stage III disease after surgery.

The remaining 20 patients were assigned to stage III prior to operation.

The postoperative revision of tumor stages and the assignment of patients to stage III was done with about equal frequency for all cell types except small cell

Table 13. Postoperative stage revision by tumor histology

	Preop. I	Postop. I/II	Postop. III	Change in %
Squamous cell	123	93	30	24.4
Adeno	35	28	7	25.0
Small cell	12	2	10	83.0
Other	16	11	5	31.0
	186	134	52	

carcinoma. As Table 13 shows, an advanced tumor stage was not recognized preoperatively in about 25% of squamous cell carcinomas and adenocarcinomas, as opposed to over 80% of small cell carcinomas.

Characteristics of Stage III Disease

Patients with stage III cancers constitute a very diverse group in which local tumor extent, advanced lymphatic spread, distant metastases, or various combinations of these factors are predominant. It is essential, therefore, that cases assigned to this stage, which often are borderline in terms of operability, be analyzed in greater detail. For this purpose we shall apply the subscripts defined previously. The stage III cases listed in Table 14 are subdivided according to tumor histology.

As the Table shows, an advanced *local tumor extent* was the most frequent basis for the diagnosis of stage III disease, combined in some cases with extrapulmonary lymph node metastases and in a few cases with hematogenous metastases.

In the absence of clinical symptoms, the invasive tendencies of a lung carcinoma are very difficult to evaluate before surgery, and preoperative staging may involve considerable error, especially when the tumor is central in origin. On the other hand, the majority of stage III cases with tracheobronchial and paratracheal lymph node involvement in our series were identified as soon as mediastinoscopy was performed.

Critical Appraisal of the TNM Systems

The definitions of the TNM system for lung carcinomas as stated in the UICC recommendations valid from 1973 to 1978 are formulated so as to provide a basis for the *clinical* staging of disease. But from a surgical standpoint, it should also be possible to make a postoperative histopathologic classification of a specific lesion that is found. It appears essential that the additional information gained from inspection of the operative site and from histopathologic evaluation of the resected tissue be documented in a simple form. The current UICC classification for malignant tumors gives consideration to this requirement by

Table 14

Squamous cell carcinomas		
$T3_{br}$ N0/1 M0	(Tumor < 2 cm from the carina)	4
$T3_{m}$ N0/1 M0	(Mediastinal invasion, 2 × aorta)	5
$T3_{pc}$ N0/1 M0	(Pericardial invasion, 2 × pericardial carcinosis)	4
$T3_{th}$ N0/1 M0	(Chest wall invasion)	1
$T3_{v}$ N0/1 M0	(Invasion of central pulmonary vessels incl. left atrium)	2
T1/2 $N2_{tb}$ M0	(Positive tracheobronchial nodes)	9
T1/2 N0/1 M1 PUL	(Pulmonary metastases, 1 × same, 2 × different lobes)	3
$T3_{br}$ $N2_{tb}$ M0		1
$T3_{m}$ $N2_{tb}$ M0		4
$T3_{th}$ $N2_{tb}$ M0		2
$T3_{pc}$ $N2_{tb}$ M0		2
$T3_{v}$ $N2_{m}$ M0		1
T2 $N2_{tb}$ M1 PUL		1
	Total	39
Adenocarcinomas		
$T3_{br}$ N1 M0		1
$T3_{m}$ N1 M0	(1 × Aorta, 1 × esophagus)	3
$T3_{pc}$ N1 M0		1
T2 $N2_{m}$ M0		2
T2 N1 M1 PUL	(Metastasis in same lobes)	2
T3 $N2_{tb}$ M1 PUL		1
T2 $N2_{m}$ M1 H/LYM	(Metastases in brain and contralateral nodes)	2
	Total	12
Small cell carcinomas		
$T3_{m}$ N0/1 M0		3
T1/2 $N2_{m}$ M0		3
$T3_{m}$ $N2_{tb}$ M0		4
$T3_{pc}$ $N2_{tb}$ M1 H	(Skeleton)	1
$T3_{pc}$ N1 M0		1
	Total	12
Other histologies		
$T3_{th}$ N0 M0		3
$T3_{v}$ N1 M0		1
T2 $N2_{tb}$ M0		1
$T3_{pc}$ $N2_{tb}$ M0		1
$T3_{pc}$ $N2_{tb}$ M1 H		1
$T3_{br}$ $N2_{tb}$ M1 PUL		1
	Total	8

recommending that clinical staging be followed by postoperative TNM staging after surgical resection is accomplished. The reliability of clinical staging is stated in terms of certainty grades C1 through C3 according to the extensiveness of the evaluation. Nevertheless, the latest UICC and AJCCS versions of the TNM classification continue to use definitions that allow for multiple interpretations.

The T Categories

TIS (carcinoma in situ), T0 (no evidence of primary tumor), and TX (tumor cannot be assessed) do not require further interpretation.

T1 is applied to tumors with a maximum diameter of 3 cm that are surrounded by lung and intact visceral pleura and do not reach or infiltrate the orifice of a lobar bronchus. This group is comprised mainly of peripheral lung tumors. Based on preoperative radiographs alone, it cannot always be determined whether a small carcinoma has crossed a lobar fissure to involve an adjacent lobe (Fig. 4a–c). With this limitation, T1 is unambiguously defined for both clinical and surgical requirements.

T2 designates tumors that either are more than 3 cm in diameter or produce atelectasis or poststenotic pneumonitis because of their central location. The tumor must be located at least 2 cm distal to the carina, and there must be no pleural effusion. Atelectasis must involve less than an entire lung.

The AJCCS version of the TNM system expressly mentions invasion of the visceral pleura. This more detailed formulation is adopted in the English text of the 1978 UICC rules and finally in the German text of the TNM Atlas published in 1985. Unfortunately, such subtle gradations cannot be clearly recognized on radiographs (Fig. 6), even when computed tomography is used. Only direct inspection and histologic examination can reliably establish the extent of disease. With small peripheral carcinomas, there is a tendency to assign a more favorable clinical stage than is actually present. The aforementioned possibility

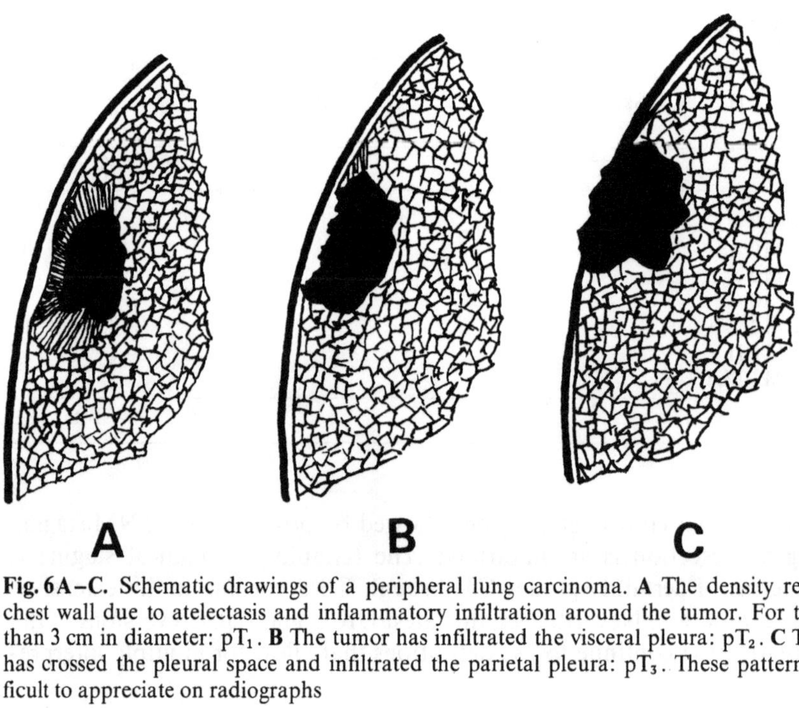

Fig. 6A–C. Schematic drawings of a peripheral lung carcinoma. **A** The density reaches the chest wall due to atelectasis and inflammatory infiltration around the tumor. For tumor less than 3 cm in diameter: pT_1. **B** The tumor has infiltrated the visceral pleura: pT_2. **C** The tumor has crossed the pleural space and infiltrated the parietal pleura: pT_3. These patterns are difficult to appreciate on radiographs

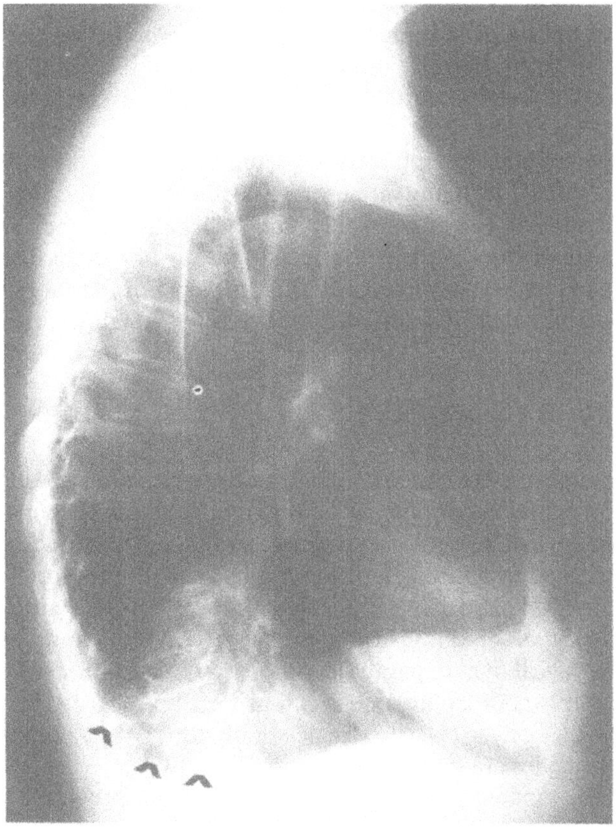

Fig. 7. Pleural effusion in the TNM classification: Always T_3? The lateral chest radiograph of this 63-year-old man (S. E.) shows segmental pneumonitis of the right lower lobe associated with a squamous cell carcinoma that is obstructing the lower lobe. The posterobasal effusion does not contain malignant cells. The visceral pleura is intact: $pT_2N_1M_0$ (stage II disease). The patient survived 3 years. Autopsy showed recurrent and metastatic cancer

of translobar tumor growth, though not specifically mentioned in any of the TNM rules, must be included in the T2 category because, in the presence of a normal pleura-lined fissure, this type of growth necessarily penetrates the visceral pleura.

In our opinion the prognostic importance of a pleural effusion, which automatically classifies a tumor as T3 in all current TNM systems, requires further differentiation. Especially with advanced cancers, pleural effusion may reflect tumor extension to the pleural space as well as lymphatic or hematogenous metastasis to the pleura. But pleural effusion may also occur in association with tumor-related bronchial stenosis and poststenotic pneumonitis even when carcinoma is not demonstrated, and so its presence is not always an absolute contraindication to surgery (Fig. 7). This point is not taken into account in current TNM rules.

T3 encompasses all local findings that go beyond the criteria of T2. Thus, from a surgical standpoint it is necessary to define the T3 category in more precise terms, because it includes patterns of disease that should be evaluated differently with regard to their resectability. A carcinoma that is closer than 2 cm to the carina or a tumor that causes atelectasis of an entire lung is more likely to be resectable completely than tumors that involve the esophagus or the myocardium. In many situations that meet all the criteria of T3 cancer, surgical treatment is both possible and rational, as for example in cases of circumscribed chest wall invasion, infiltration of the pericardium and atrium, or tumors that closely approach the carina. With limitations, a number of T3 lesions are amenable to curative or at least questionably curative surgical resection.

The N Categories

Noninvasive methods are of questionable value in establishing the N status of a bronchial carcinoma. It is apparent that enlargements of intrathoracic lymph nodes can be demonstrated by radiologic techniques, especially tomography of the mediastinum, esophagography with fluoroscopy, and computed tomography [126, 161, 223]. But unless there is concomitant clinical or radiologic evidence of organ invasion arising from the lymph nodes, such as recurrent laryngeal nerve paralysis or obvious disruption of the esophageal contour, lymph node enlargement can at best be regarded as *suspicious* for metastasis [123]. Conversely, the absence of obvious lymphadenopathy does not prove that the nodes are free of metastatic cancer [35].

Computed tomography of the chest can provide a three times higher sensitivity (90%) than conventional tomography in the detection of enlarged lymph nodes [99a]. However, a literature survey by Koenig et al. (1984) indicates a wide range of sensitivity rates for the CT method, with better rates reported for enlarged tracheobronchial nodes than for hilar nodes. Reports on the specificity of the method also vary considerably, so that the presence of enlarged nodes on computed tomograms is not in itself pathognomonic for nodal metastasis. On the other hand, lymph nodes that appear normal on CT scans are rarely involved by metastasis.

Isotope enhancement appears to be a promising source of information for selected tumor histologies. Isotope accumulation is fairly nonspecific, however, occurring both in inflammatory lesions and in neoplasms, and the technique has not yet been adequately tested in routine clinical use [5, 247].

According to a study by Broughton et al. [42a], gallium scanning with conventional recording is useful for demonstrating lymphatic spread in selected patients, although it is not recommended as a routine investigation.

Mediastinoscopy is a far more powerful diagnostic tool that enables the physician to evaluate grossly and histologically the important central lymph nodes of the paratracheal and tracheobronchial region.

The designation *N0* is applied to cases in which there is no demonstrable metastatic involvement of regional lymph nodes. In a surgical population, N0 is applied to cases in which histologic examination of the surgical specimen and

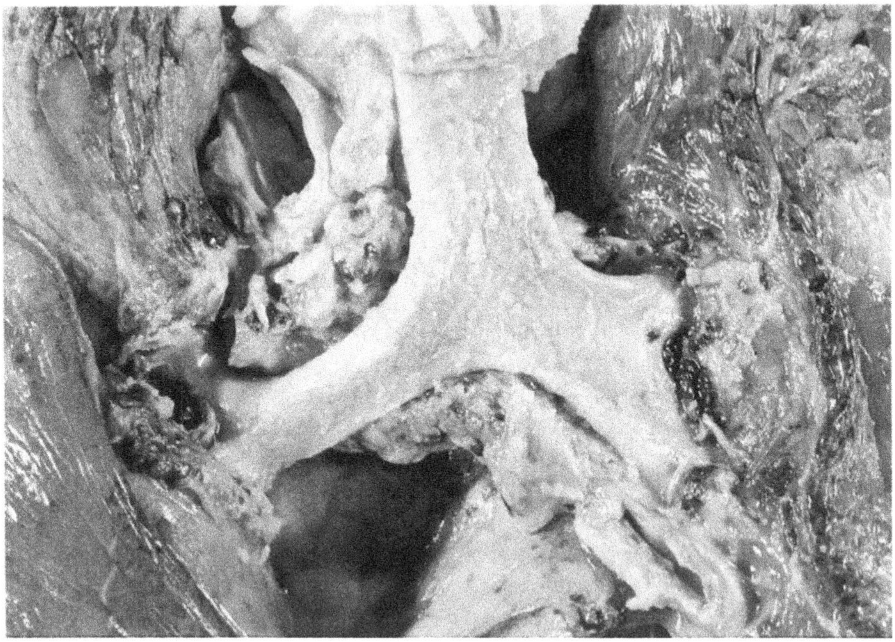

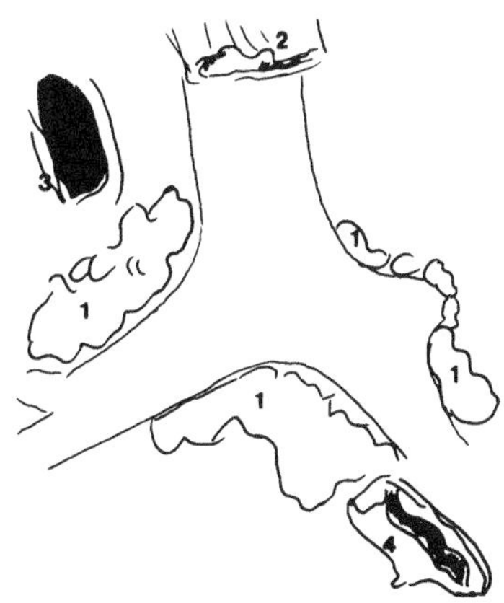

Fig. 8. Dorsal view of a specimen of the tracheal bifurcation demonstrating the small distance between right upper lobe bronchus and trachea and illustrating the problem of distinction between hilar (N_1) and mediastinal (N_2) metastatic nodes on the right. *1*, lymph nodes; *2*, esophagus; *3* aorta; *4* main pulmonary artery

resected extrapulmonary lymph nodes shows no evidence of lymphatic metastasis.

N 1 denotes the involvement of lymph nodes in the *peribronchial or ipsilateral hilar region*, including the direct invasion of adjacent nodes. In practice, a lesion can be classified as N 1 only by operative means. Differentiation from N 2 is occasionally difficult because there is no clear anatomic dividing line between the hilar and mediastinal nodes. Especially in the area of the right hilus, this distinction tends to be somewhat arbitrary [83] because the extrapulmonary portion of the main bronchus is only a few millimeters long (Fig. 8). Evaluation is less difficult on the left side, where an extrapulmonary segment of main bronchus about 4 cm long courses posterior to the great vessels.

N 2, in both the English and German TNM versions, is defined as the involvement of *mediastinal* lymph nodes. The text of the AJCCS [48, 230] modifies this formulation with its definition of M 1, in which involvement of the *contralateral hilar* lymph nodes is considered to be equivalent to distant metastasis. This makes allowance for the fact that resection is feasible when there is mediastinal lymph node involvement on the side where the tumor is located, but that surgery is contraindicated by nodal metastasis on the opposite side [164, 227]. The German version allows a similar interpretation, because the N definitions are listed under the heading Regional Lymph Nodes, and it can be argued that lymph nodes outside a hemithorax are no longer regional. Because metastasis to contralateral lymph nodes ordinarily precludes operative treatment, there is little point in debating this issue. In certain cases, however, palliative operations are worthwhile despite known lymphatic metastases on the contralateral side. We have assigned such patients to the group $M\,1_{(lym)}$.

With regard to future development of the TNM system, it would be desirable from a surgical standpoint to have a clearer distinction drawn between ipsilateral and contralateral lymph node metastases.

The distinction between tumor confined within the capsule of the lymph nodes and tumor that has penetrated the nodal capsule, to which Hermanek and Gall [128 a] ascribe prognostic significance, is easily accomplished by the addition of a subscript.

The M Categories

While the M classification of lung carcinoma appears to be a simple matter, we again find that various interpretations are possible in practice.

M 0 means that there is no evidence of distant metastases. Aside from the fact that this classification in no way assures the absence of distant metastases, this definition is unambiguous.

M 1 is used when distant metastases are known to be present, regardless of the mode (lymphatic or hematogenous) of tumor spread. By this definition, distant metastases are cancerous lymph nodes outside the bounds of the ipsilateral region [164] and metastases in extrapulmonary organs. *Pulmonary* metastases require further clarification. Earlier UICC definitions make no specific reference to pulmonary metastases from primary lung carcinoma. The AJCCS version interprets metastatic lesions of the *contralateral* lung as distant metastases, excluding ipsilateral metastases. The latest version of the UICC classification takes pulmonary metastases into account by recommending that the subscript "pul" be added to designate them, but it does not address the question of ipsilateral versus contralateral involvement. The problem is complicated by the fact that carcinomas may arise multicentrically. According to Spencer [322], carcinomas occurring in different pulmonary lobes may both be primary neoplasms even if their histologies are the same. We believe that multiple carcinomatous foci reflect a highly virulent disease process regardless of the side of their occurrence, and we therefore feel that pulmonary metastases always warrant a classification of M 1, particularly since existing classification systems offer no alternative in situations of this kind (cf. p. 25).

Stage Grouping

The grouping of various TNM combinations into stages is based on the concept that certain patterns of disease imply similar prognoses. Prior to 1978 the staging system of the UICC recognized the following three stages of lung cancer based on the TNM classification:

Stage I:	T0/TX, N1, M0
	T1, N0/N1, M0
	T2, N0, M0
Stage II:	T2, N1, M0
Stage III:	Any T3, any N2, any M1

The most recent version of the UICC system [340] subdivides stage I cases into Ia, without lymph node metastases, and Ib, with lymph node metastases, provided the extent of disease is limited to T0/T1, N1, M0. Stage Ib disease must be diagnosed surgically, and so this classification is not relevant to pretherapeutic staging. Indeed, experience in surgically treated patients raises doubt as to whether it is appropriate to place cases with lymph node involvement and a small primary tumor into the relatively favorable stage I category. Salzer [286, 287] classifies the combination T1, N1, M0 as stage II, and so does Naef [236]. Shields [302] also questions whether lymph node involvement is compatible with a diagnosis of stage I disease.

None of the patients in this study had the criteria of stage Ib disease or a T1, N1, M0 lesion. Without exception, tumors with associated lymph node metastases were either larger than 3 cm in diameter or failed to satisfy other T1 criteria.

The current version of the UICC classification introduces a stage IV category that is applied to all patients with distant metastases, without regard for local or regional tumor spread. As mentioned earlier, we classified our M1 patients, all of whom had pulmonary metastases, as having stage III disease.

Stage Grouping as of February 1986

Occult cancer:	TX, N0, M0
Stage Ia:	T1, N0, M0
	T2, N0, M0
Stage Ib:	T0/T1, N1, M0
Stage II:	T2, N1, M0
Stage III:	T3, N0/N1, M0
	Any T, N2, M0
Stage IV:	Any T, any N, M1

Chapter 3

Preoperative Diagnosis – Selection for Operation

Oncologic Diagnosis

It is generally agreed that the surgical resection of a lung carcinoma can be life-prolonging or curative only if the tumor is completely eradicated. This means that the lesion itself must be resectable, and that regional metastases either must be absent or must be removable at the time of tumor resection. Accordingly, the goal of preoperative diagnosis in the cancer patient is to determine whether these criteria are met in the individual surgical candidate.

With advances in medical technology, the physician has a growing number of investigative methods at his disposal. However, there are several factors which place relatively narrow constraints on the number and type of investigations that may be performed routinely. One is the physical and psychological tolerance of the patient. Another is the loss of time and delay in therapy, which we believe is an urgent consideration. Finally there is the financial factor, which is becoming increasingly important in the current socioeconomic setting.

For these reasons, the procedures used to make a diagnosis, stage the tumor, and assess its operability must be selected with a view toward maximizing the efficiency of the evaluation while minimizing the risk to the patient. It is also essential that investigations be performed in a logical sequence. If operability still has not been established at the conclusion of the basic work-up, additional special investigations may be performed.

By the start of the present study, a program had already been outlined for the oncologic evaluation of patients considered to be surgical candidates. Because almost all patients were originally admitted to the Basel University Clinic through the Department of Internal Medicine, mainly the Pneumologic Division, interdisciplinary cooperation was necessary. The same applies to innovations that were introduced during the course of the study.

Of course, the sequence of investigation presented below is not ideal for all cases, and clinical findings that are noted on admission have to be considered. For example, suspicious findings on palpation of the liver would warrant the exclusion or confirmation of hepatic metastases as a primary part of the work-up. It also should be noted that the sequence of investigation is designed for patients who appear functionally able to tolerate surgery based on initial clinical evaluation.

The standard procedure for the evaluation of candidates for elective lung cancer surgery is shown in Table 15.

Table 15. Sequence of oncologic investigations

Routine investigations	Special investigations
1. Radiologic diagnosis	
a) Chest radiographs in two planes	Spot films
b) Barium fluoroscopy of esophagus	Tomograms
c) Skeletal radiographs (until June, 1974)	Pleural aspiration (cytology)
2. Bronchoscopy	
a) Rigid bronchoscopy	
b) Fiberoptic bronchoscopy Biopsies, washings, brushings	
3. Laboratory investigations	
a) Sputum cytology (at least 3 samples)	
b) Bone marrow biopsy (until Dec., 1975)[a]	
c) Hepatic enzymes	Further liver studies are done if values are abnormal (scanning, sonotomography)
4. Nuclear imaging	
a) Liver scan (until Dec., 1974)	Laparoscopy Needle biopsy
b) Bone scan (until July, 1974)	Spot films, tomograms Bone marrow biopsy
c) Brain scan[b] (until Dec., 1974)	
5. Cranial CT scan[b] (since 1975)	
6. Mediastinoscopy	

[a] Still indicated with (suspicion of) small cell carcinoma
[b] Indicated only with (suspicion of) small cell carcinoma

Radiologic Investigations

Standard Chest Radiographs

Radiographs of the chest in two planes are basic to pulmonary diagnosis. In the great majority of cases the sagittal chest radiograph raises the initial suspicion of a lung tumor, whether in the setting of a general examination or in the symptomatic patient. A lateral chest radiograph is also necessary, not only for the assessment of surgical candidates but also for the investigation of virtually any form of pulmonary disease [45, 49, 74, 198, 247, 301] (Fig. 9a + b).

During preoperative planning, chest radiographs combined with endoscopy can localize the tumor with a fairly high degree of accuracy. According to Miller [221] and Oeser [246], lesions located in aerated lung parenchyma can be detected and localized down to a critical diameter of 5–10 mm. Centrally located

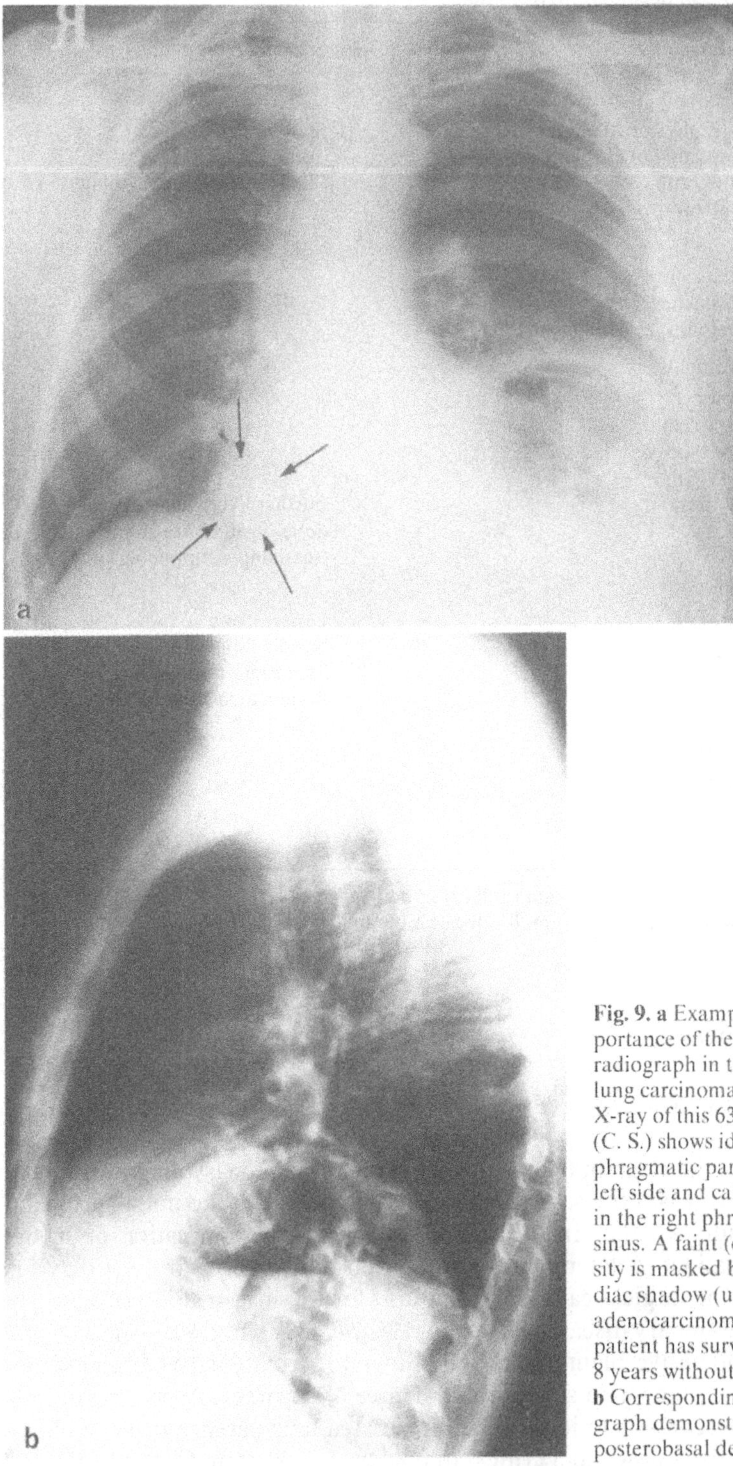

Fig. 9. a Example of the importance of the lateral chest radiograph in the diagnosis of lung carcinoma. The PA chest X-ray of this 63-year-old man (C. S.) shows idiopathic diaphragmatic paralysis on the left side and calcified residue in the right phrenicocostal sinus. A faint (overlooked) density is masked by the right cardiac shadow (undifferentiated adenocarcinoma $T_2N_0M_0$; patient has survived almost 8 years without symptoms). **b** Corresponding lateral radiograph demonstrating a large posterobasal density

tumors of that size cannot be directly visualized on X-rays, although secondary radiographic changes of the lung such as overinflation from partial bronchial obstruction can call attention to their presence [70]. With lesions that cause complete obstruction, the presence of atelectasis (segmental, lobar, or total) can provide secondary radiographic evidence of tumor.

Besides demonstrating the size and anatomic location of the tumor, the standard chest films supply information on possible chest wall infiltration, phrenic nerve involvement with elevation of the diaphragm, and pleural effusion. Widening of the mediastinum by inflammatory or metastatic lymph node enlargement, destruction of bone, and additional nodular lesions of the parenchyma can provide the basis for further, more specialized investigations.

It was not until the conclusion of the present study that computed tomography became available for the evaluation of bronchial carcinoma. Today it is a routine diagnostic study, and generally we include the epigastric region in CT scans. Computed tomography has helped to narrow the indications for mediastinoscopy (p. 28) without increasing the rate of exploratory thoracotomies.

Standard chest radiographs are not only useful for tumor diagnosis; they can also furnish important information on the patient's cardiorespiratory status, diffuse or localized emphysema, right or left ventricular enlargement, tuberculous lesions, etc.

As a rule, we required radiographs that were no more than two weeks old at the time of thoracotomy.

Fluoroscopy

Fluoroscopy supplements the static films taken at full inspiration by allowing an accurate assessment of diaphragmatic motion, the displacement of a peripheral lesion toward the chest wall, and shifting fluid levels in the case of pleural effusion.

Contrast Imaging of the Esophagus

In all patients chest fluoroscopy was supplemented by a contrast study of esophageal function and contour. Displacement of the esophagus by a tumor or enlarged posterior mediastinal nodes implies a need for extensive surgery, while a discontinuity in the contour of the mucosa is a sign of direct or metastatic invasion that would contraindicate surgery [61].

Skeletal Radiographs

Given the frequency of bone metastases from bronchial carcinoma, it seemed reasonable to obtain routine X-ray films of the cranium, spine, pelvis, and extremities [55].

Most data on the modes of lung cancer metastasis are derived from unselected populations in which advanced tumor stages predominate, or from autopsy findings in patients who died from lung carcinoma [201, 232]. According to Hansen et al. [110], routine skeletal radiographs have a disappointing yield in the screening of lung cancer populations. Even in a series of inoperable patients, the yield from the method was far lower than from bone marrow biopsy. This is consistent with our experience that no patient was excluded from operation primarily on the basis of *radiologic* evidence of bone metastases. This led us to discontinue routine skeletal radiography in mid-1974. Skeletal radiographs are still useful, however, and are ordered whenever bone scans raise the suspicion of skeletal metastasis.

Bronchoscopy

Bronchoscopy, like chest radiography, is a basic modality in the diagnosis of central as well as peripheral bronchial carcinoma and hence is performed early in the course of the preoperative evaluation. There are cases in which the suspicion and diagnosis of bronchial carcinoma was based not on chest radiographs, but on bronchoscopy performed in a patient with cough or hemoptysis. In contrast to the X-ray film, which, strictly speaking, can only raise the *suspicion* of tumor, bronchoscopy permits the direct visualization of endobronchial neoplasms and the detection of other tumors by evidence of bronchial compression or displacement of the cartilages.

Marsh et al. [207] state that endoscopy with the rigid bronchoscope can yield a definitive result in one-third of patients examined. The introduction of flexible bronchoscopy [147], which extends the range of vision to the subsegmental bronchi, has made the visual detection of neoplasms more frequent, and above all has provided a means of collecting histologic and cytologic specimens with a positive yield in excess of 70% [207].

Bronchoscopy, like radiography, has uses which go beyond the localization and classification of tumors. It enables the physician to evaluate the tracheobronchial architecture (evidence of collapse, check-valve syndrome) and the condition of the airway mucosa (acute or chronic bronchitis). In the presence of abnormal bronchial secretions, bronchoscopy allows the gathering of material for specific bacteriologic testing. It also is possible to assess vocal cord status as the instrument traverses the larynx. The demonstration of recurrent laryngeal nerve paralysis can be an important and time-saving aid to preoperative diagnosis.

We agree with Watson et al. [352] that the surgeon who is to perform the definitive resection should have an opportunity to view the tracheobronchial tree through the bronchoscope. This will provide the degree of experience necessary for making decisions regarding, say, the extirpation of a tumor in proximity to the trachea or the feasibility of a sleeve resection. Because virtually all patients underwent mediastinoscopy, "surgical" endoscopy with the fiberoptic bronchoscope was performed in the intubated and anesthetized patient and so did not pose an additional stress.

Laboratory Investigations

Sputum Cytology

The collection of sputum for cytologic evaluation is one of the most effective methods available for the qualitative diagnosis of lung carcinoma. However, the diagnostic yield depends on proper collection by the well instructed patient [192, 282, 323]. The likelihood of positive sputum cytology in a patient with bronchial carcinoma is greatest when morning sputum is raised by intense coughing after saliva has been expectorated. The yield increases with the number of specimens examined. The morning after bronchoscopy has proved to be a particularly favorable time for sputum collection [218].

On occasion, preliminary antibiotic therapy may be necessary to relieve inflammatory obstruction before positive sputum can be obtained [73].

Bone Marrow Biopsy

The purpose of bone marrow studies in preoperative diagnosis is to exclude a form of occult metastasis that is common with bronchial carcinoma, or to confirm the presence of such metastasis as a contraindication to surgery. Routine iliac crest biopsies were taken in all patients prior to 1975, regardless of whether carcinoma had been histologically proved or classified. But with a yield of less than 5% for all carcinomas and less than 2% for non-small cell carcinomas – a figure confirmed by Hansen et al. [110] – continuation of these biopsies could no longer be justified. Since 1975 we perform bone marrow biopsies only in patients with undifferentiated small cell carcinoma [108].

Hepatic Enzymes

The only serum analysis that may be considered relevant to diagnosis of metastatic disease is the assay of hepatic enzymes (SGOT, SGPT, alkaline phosphatase, gamma GT, leucine aminopeptidase). With an elevation of one or more of these enzymes, a search should be made for hepatic metastases.

Cranial Computed Tomography (EMI Scan)

Following the development and widespread use of computed tomography, which was first used in craniocerebral investigations, it was natural to apply CT as a screening method for metastases in lung cancer patients. Since 1975 we have used CT screening in patients with neurologic symptoms and in all patients with small cell carcinomas. (Thoracic and abdominal CT, which now are clinically established, were not available for the patients admitted to this study.)

Nuclear Imaging

Liver Scanning

Nonselective liver scans were a routine preoperative study during the period 1973–1974. Because no patient who lacked clinical symptoms (hepatomegaly, jaundice, ascites) or elevated serum hepatic enzymes had an abnormal liver scan, the procedure was subsequently removed from the list of routine investigations. A study by Guttierez et al. [105] confirms that the sensitivity of the method is too low to justify its routine use. In 47 patients who died within 10 weeks of the examination, autopsy showed a 34% rate of false-negative diagnoses and a 4% rate of false positives.

Bone Scanning

In July, 1974, radionuclide bone scanning replaced skeletal radiography as a routine diagnostic investigation. This decision was based on the relatively high efficacy of the method [105, 139, 232]. Metastasis-related osteolytic foci less than 1.5 cm in diameter are not detectable on X-rays, but they are visible on bone scans. The concentration of radionuclide in bone is not specific for metastasis, however, and also occurs in inflammatory and posttraumatic lesions. Thus, abnormal uptakes were always clarified by skeletal spot radiographs or tomograms, and in doubtful cases by biopsy if the suspicious area was accessible.

Brain Scanning

Before the advent of computed tomography in craniocerebral diagnosis, we used brain scans for the metastatic screening of all patients with small cell undifferentiated carcinoma. Afterward the procedure was reserved for patients who had clinical symptoms of neurologic involvement.

Mediastinoscopy

In November, 1972, we adopted mediastinoscopy as a *routine* investigation in our lung cancer patients. Of 206 patients, 20 did not undergo mediastinoscopy – 11 in the period from February to October, 1972, and 9 during the remainder of the study (Table 16). In these latter patients, mediastinoscopy was withheld in five cases because the indication for operation was palliative (one operation was an emergency procedure for acute hemoptysis). In four cases the examination was not done because the risk was felt to be prohibitive (two had had previous mediastinal radiation, and two had upper inflow stasis). Later we learned that the risk of uncontrolled hemorrhage is not excessive in the presence of in-

Table 16. Thoracotomy without mediastinoscopy

a) before November, 1972 (see text)

Pat.	Histology preop.	Histology postop.	Operation	Lymphnode metastases	Follow up
B.H., m.	SCC	SCC	Explor.	mediast.	† 6 weeks
G.R., m.	Squam.	Squam.	Explor.	hilar	† 23 months
H.A., m.	Ø	SCC	Explor.	mediast.	† 7 months
H.B., m.	Squam.	Squam.	Lobect.	Ø	surv. over 10 years
J.W., m.	Squam.	Squam.	Pneumonect.	hilar	† 10 years (no recurr.)
K.K., f.	Ø	Adeno	Lobect.	Ø	† 18 months
L.P., m.	Squam.	Squam.	Pneumonect.	Ø	† 5 months
M.R., m.	Papilloma	Squam.	Explor.	hilar	† 8 months
P.E., m.	Squam.	Squam.	Bilobect.	hilar	† 16 months
S.M., m.	Ø	Squam.	Pneumonect.	mediast.	† 50 months (no recurr.)
S.W., m.	Ø	Squam.	Pneumonect.	hilar	operative death (pos. nodes opposit mediastinum)

b) in palliative interventions or other contraindications

Pat.	Histology preop.	Histology postop.	Reason for palliation	Operation	LN	Follow up
B.C., m.	Ø	SCC	SVCO	Shunt	med.	† 16 months
B.E., m.	Ø	SCC	SVCO	Explor.	med.	† 4 months
R.L., f.	Ø	Squam.	former Hodgkin radiotherapy	Lobect.	interlobar	† 28 months
R.E., f.	Ø	LCC	abscess	Lobect.	Ø	† 24 months
S.A., m.	Squam.	Squam.	abscess	Lobect.	Ø	† 20 months
S.R., m.	unclassified		radiother. sp. sulcus syndrom	Lobect.	Ø	† 8 months
S.P., m.	Squam.	Squam.	abscess	Pneumonect.	Hil.	† 6 months
E.H., m.	LCC	LCC	hemoptysis	Pneumonect.	hil.	† 6 years (recurr.)
W.U., m.	Adeno	Adeno	brain metastasis debulking-surgery	Lobect.	hil.	† 17 months

SCC: small cell carcinoma
LCC: large cell carcinoma
Squam.: squamous cell carc.
SVCO: superior v. cava obstruction
†: death

flow stasis, and that mediastinoscopy is an excellent means of establishing the cause [63]. The procedure is more problematic in the late phase after radiation therapy, when the dissection of tissue layers must be forced.

As an operative procedure that requires general anesthesia, mediastinoscopy for the staging of lung cancer remains controversial, and the debate between its proponents and opponents will probably continue.

The publications of Salzer [288], Delarue and Strasberg [61], Specht [321], Pearson [260], and Maassen and Greschuchna [202] have convinced us of the effectiveness of the procedure. All these authors report an increase in resection rates and a decrease in the rate of exploratory thoracotomies from 30%–40% to approximately 5% of all operations.

Twenty thoracotomies that were performed without prior mediastinoscopy in our series effectively form a control group that is important despite its small size. In 6 of these cases (30%) the operation had to be terminated as a simple thoracotomy. Of 186 patients who were selected for mediastinoscopy, only 10 (6.4%) underwent exploratory thoracotomy. As the graph in Fig. 2 shows (p. 4), the incidence of nonresective thoracotomies has further declined since 1975, apparently as a result of increasing experience with the examination technique and a declining rate of false-negative findings.

This alone could not justify the routine use of mediastinoscopy were it not for the fact that the procedure carries a low morbidity and mortality, especially since patients with suspected carcinoma that is not pathologically confirmed and is later excluded by surgery also are candidates for the examination.

It is not surprising that the large volume of literature on mediastinoscopy includes reports of complications and even deaths relating to the procedure.

In the 532 mediastinoscopies performed for various indications at the Cardiothoracic Surgical Unit of Basel University Hospital from 1972 through 1981, no fatal complications occurred, and no other complications arose that necessitated thoracotomy [119]. Two patients developed a pneumothorax that was managed by transmediastinal drainage. Six mediastinoscopies were associated with significant hemorrhage caused by injury to the pulmonary artery or azygos vein. In each case the hemorrhage was satisfactorily controlled through the endoscope with a maximum blood loss of 400 ml. One patient with bronchogenic carcinoma was a poor surgical candidate, having undergone previous mediastinoscopy followed by radiation to the mediastinum. The right mainstem bronchus of this patient was bluntly penetrated (cf. [260]), but the lesion healed spontaneously after prolonged drainage and antibiotic therapy. Two patients suffered irreversible recurrent laryngeal nerve paralysis. It should be noted that complications become less frequent as experience is gained [163]; hence the sporadic use of mediastinoscopy is not advised because of the excessive risk and the relatively low yield [117].

The value of systematic mediastinoscopic exploration lies not just in the avoidance of needless thoracotomies, which, according to Akovbiantz [4], has a mortality rate averaging 10%. Another important aspect of the procedure is its ability to provide broader insight into the pattern of the lymphatic spread of lung carcinomas [100, 101, 120, 198, 279, 341].

According to collective statistics published by Ashbaugh in 1970 [12], 9 fatal complications occurred in a total of more than 9500 examinations (=0.09%). Stanulla und Duerschmid [328] report a 2.9% incidence of complications in 2276 mediastinoscopies, one of which necessitated a thoracotomy. None had a fatal outcome.

Clagett [53] states that mediastinoscopies should be performed only by examiners who are intimately familiar with tracheobronchial anatomy and are able to manage any complications that may arise. With the same proviso, and noting that the complication rate falls as experience is gained, in 1972 Laurenzi et al. [189] recommend on behalf of the American Thoracic Society (Committee on Therapy) that mediastinoscopy be utilized more widely in the investigation of benign and malignant processes.

Between the extremes of advocating the routine use of mediastinoscopy [3, 8, 14, 81, 182, 203, 242, 260–262] for preoperative staging or as a preliminary to radiotherapy or chemotherapy [95, 96] and rejecting the procedure entirely [315], there are some authors who recommend a selective approach. For example, Guinn et al. [104], Hutchinson and Mills [144], Acosta and Manfredi [2], and Peace and Price [259] suggest that mediastinoscopy be performed when there is widening of the mediastinum, the tumor is centrally located, or the histologic diagnosis is undifferentiated carcinoma. Sealy [295] also speaks of a large number of "unproductive" operations (with negative metastatic findings) and recommends that suspicious radiologic findings be made a criterion for the use of mediastinoscopy. Lacquet [185, 186] states that the procedure is not indicated in patients with peripheral coin lesions of the lung. In response to a survey taken by Paris et al. [252], 14 of 43 surgeons in the United States and Europe stated that they always used mediastinoscopy, and 12 said that they rarely used it. The remaining 17 stated that they used mediastinoscopy in patients with suspicious radiologic findings.

Other authors point to the limited efficacy of the procedure in evaluations of the left subaortic lymph nodes and advise the more extensive procedure of anterior mediastinotomy [24, 159, 215, 270, 329].

All suggestions for limiting patient selection ignore the fact that mediastinoscopy is essential to the diagnosis of contralateral metastasis. Indirect methods such as nuclear imaging [5, 274, 345] and computed tomography [126, 161, 223] are incapable of distinguishing between cancerous and inflammatory lymph node enlargement, or detecting metastases in nodes that are not enlarged (Fig. 10).

Efficacy of Specific Methods in the Diagnosis of Carcinoma

A basic goal of preoperative diagnosis is to confirm the carcinoma in qualitative terms. In presenting the distribution of cell types in the present series, we noted that one-third of the patients were operated on without histologic or cytologic proof of malignant disease.

If the diagnosis of carcinoma was not confirmed preoperatively in 69 cases, this does not necessarily mean that the diagnostic work-up was inadequate. Also, one must be careful about making comparisons with series that are not purely surgical, as the proportion of advanced carcinomas in such series tends to be high [25].

Most peripheral carcinomas, many of which were small, were not verified histologically until resection was carried out. Sixty-six patients (presumed to have lung carcinoma) were diagnosed preoperatively as having clinical stage I disease.

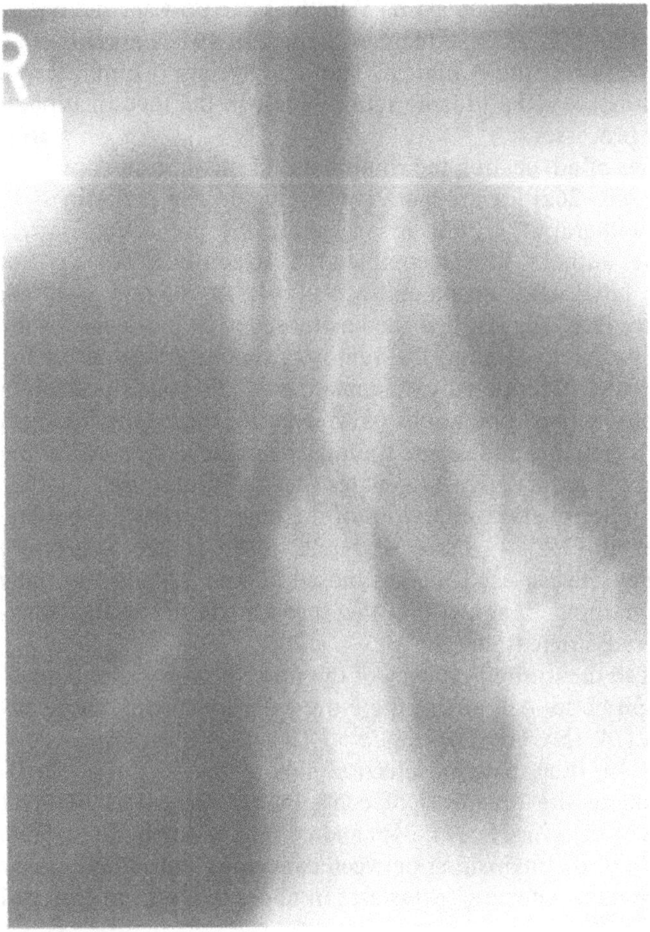

Fig. 10. Tomogram of a radiologically normal mediastinum with bilateral paratracheal and tracheobronchial lymph node metastases from an adenocarcinoma (detected at mediastinoscopy) in a 43-year-old-woman ($pT_2N_2M_{1\ lym}$; adjuvant lobectomy, chemotherapy; patient survived 24 months)

Certainly, we could have made greater use of percutaneous needle biopsy [14]. But the use of a cutting needle to obtain a core of parenchyma for histologic examination raises the danger of various complications such as pneumothorax, hematothorax, and hemoptysis, whose risks are far from negligible. The lower-risk fine-needle aspiration biopsy is useful only for cytologic evaluation. Moreover, a negative biopsy can rarely be taken as proof of the absence of carcinoma, so usually it is not worthwhile to demand biopsy confirmation of a suspected carcinoma [31, 62, 106, 132, 162, 249, 272, 348].

Comparing specific investigations with regard to the frequency of positive results, we find that sputum cytology has by far the highest yield. With tumors that are visible within the bronchial tree, selective biopsy is a reliable means of

Table 17. Efficacy of specific methods in the preoperative diagnosis of lung carcinoma

Method	Patients with pos. result in only one method	Total positive results per method
Sputum cytology	32	76
Bronchoscopy		
Biopsy	21	47
Washing	12	43
Brushing	5	21
Fine-needle aspiration	7	10
Mediastinoscopy	3	18
1 Method positive	80	
2 Cytolog. methods positive	20	
Cytology + biopsy positive	26	
3 Methods positive	11	
Carcinoma confirmed	137	
Carcinoma not confirmed	69	
Total	206	

establishing a qualitative diagnosis of carcinoma. Table 17 compares the efficacies of the different diagnostic methods in establishing carcinoma prior to operation.

Besides the 69 patients whose carcinomas were not confirmed until operation, there were 60 patients with suspected carcinoma in whom surgery did not disclose evidence of malignant disease. Except for two organized peripheral pulmonary infarctions, all other lesions proved to require resection, and there was no operative mortality.

Function Testing

In many cases the question of whether an individual patient can tolerate a thoracotomy and a resection of the necessary extent can be answered by careful history taking, clinical examination, and simple performance tests. R. A. Smith [313] introduces a report on 1250 resections in 22 years with the words, "As far as preoperative assessment is concerned, we do very little," and with regard to function testing, "We observe the effect of a mile walk on the patient repeated several times." One carcinoma patient in 7 was operated on in this series; the resection rate (not always curative) was 97%, and mortality was 7.1%.

We are convinced that an approach of this kind inevitably leads to overestimation or underestimation of cardiorespiratory functional reserves. Today, most authorities recognize the need for instrumental function testing in candidates for pulmonary resective surgery, both to limit the operative risk and risk of disability and also to ensure that surgery is not wrongly withheld from acceptable candidates. Mountain [231] writes that "pulmonary function evaluation is mandatory before the surgical resection of lung tissue." Of course, as in oncologic evaluation, the spectrum of available investigations has become so broad that an effective selection must be made. Supplementary tests can be used to resolve doubtful cases.

From the beginning, all candidates for elective surgery were subject to a standardized program of function testing (Table 18). The thrust of this program was to confirm functional operability whenever possible by the use of differentiating studies or by preliminary therapy and reexamination.

Table 18 necessarily omits certain factors that had a significant bearing on the assessment of operability. These are the evaluation of the patient's clinical status, his general state of health, evidence of coexisting organ insufficiency, and psychologic status. The table also neglects the influence of concurrent find-

Table 18. Preoperative function tests

Pulmonary function	Hemodynamics
Bronchospirometry	
TLC (total lung capacity)	ECG Right heart catheterization during rest and exercise[a]
VC (vital capacity)	
FRC (functional residual capacity)	– Pressure measurement – Mixed venous oxygen saturation
FEV_1 (1-second forced expiratory volume)	– Calculation of cardiac output and pulmonary artery resistance
R (bronchial resistance)	
Arterial blood gas analysis	
P_aO_2 (rest/exercise and room air/100% O_2)	
If function is critically impaired:	
Differential spirometry or Ventilation-perfusion scan	Perfusion scan
If operability is still in doubt:	
THERAPY	
Antibiotics Secretolytics Bronchodilators Steroids (Positive-pressure) inhalation Physiotherapy	Digitalization
Repetition of relevant function tests:	
Definitive decision	

[a] Except in patients less than 45 years of age with no cardiac complaints, a normal ECG, and no serious impairment of pulmonary function

Table 19 [a]

Prerequisites for pneumonectomy:	
1. FEV_1	At least 2 liters At least 50% of VC
2. VC	At least 80% of normal value If less than 80% normal: Ventilation-perfusion scan At least 40% normal on the healthy side
3. Bronchial resistance R: no more than 5 cm H_2O/L/sec	
4. PAP_{mean} no more than 35 mm Hg during exercise (40 watts)	
Prerequisites for lobectomy:	
1. FEV_1	At least 40% of VC
2. VC	At least 50% of normal value
3. P_aO_2	At least 50 mm Hg

[a] After Perruchoud et al. [264], see also Heindl and Zwick [125]

ings obtained by radiography or bronchoscopy during the course of oncologic testing.

Pulmonary Function Criteria for Operability

Our criteria for the consideration of lobectomy or pneumonectomy are summarized in Table 19.

Their intent is to ensure that the patient will have a one-second forced expiratory volume (FEV_1) of at least 1 l after the operation. Taube and Konietzko showed in clinical tests that lung scans can accurately predict the postoperative FEV_1 in doubtful cases [330, 331]. They use the formula

$$FEV_{1\,(postop)} = \frac{FEV_{1\,(preop)} \times \%\ \textit{perfusion of healthy side}}{100}$$

When we applied this formula to our patients, we found a slight underestimation of the actual FEV_1 measured postoperatively.

Additional aids and suggestions for the assessment of lung function and operative risk, some in diagrammatic form, may be found in Ellison [68], Vogel et al. [347], Lockwood [196a, 196b, 197], Fischer [79], and Wassner and Timm [350].

Practical Aspects of Function Testing

The great majority of our patients were hospitalized for the preoperative work-up. This is recommended, as it enables the entire evaluation to be completed within a few days. Oncologic and function tests are conducted in parallel fashion, and the information obtained influences the further course of the evaluation. If technical or oncologic inoperability is confirmed, the patient is spared more invasive function tests. Similarly, if the patient's functional status contraindicates surgery, studies to establish technical operability may be omitted. Functional disorders that seem amenable to therapy may be treated right away without loss of time. In all cases the period of the evaluation is utilized to make standard preparations for the operation that may follow. This approach reduces the psychologic stress on the patient, allows for daily communication, and shortens the period of uncertainty about what will happen next [214].

Results of Function Testing

The functional results reported here pertain exclusively to the patients who underwent surgery (n = 206). The parameters selected were considered suitable for the characterization of operative risk in these patients, and data are given on the correlation of abnormal findings with postoperative complications, although a separate chapter is devoted to that issue.

ECG and Clinical Cardiovascular Status

Preoperative resting electrocardiograms were available for all patients. In 175 cases the history and clinical cardiovascular findings were unremarkable; 139 patients had normal ECGs. Coronary artery disease was the most frequent confirmed cardiac pathology. Eleven patients showed marked ECG evidence of prior myocardial infarction, and 16 others had chronic angina pectoris. Six patients were under treatment for significant hypertension; five had no associated ECG changes. Three patients showed evidence of cardiac valve defects, but these were unaccompanied by significant ECG abnormalities. Two of the patients had mild mitral valve insufficiency – one a mild aortic stenosis with no subjective symptoms, a normal carotid pulse, and no ECG evidence of hypertrophy.

Postoperative cardiac complications (cf. p. 69) occurred in 12 (8.6%) of the 139 patients with normal ECGs and a satisfactory cardiac status, as opposed to 8 (12%) of the remaining patients with history or clinical evidence of cardiovascular disease. This difference is not statistically significant.

Pulmonary Hemodynamics

In 19 patients the hemodynamics of the pulmonary circulation were not tested by right heart catheterization. In 13 cases this was due to technical difficulties relating to failure of passage of the catheter through a peripheral vein. If there was no serious, concomitant impairment of lung function, the examination was not forced. In six patients the urgency of surgery obviated the need for cardiac catheterization.

Four of the 187 examinations were performed at rest because the patients were unable to operate the bicycle ergometer. These patients had normal resting pressures in the pulmonary circuit.

A complete examination performed in 183 patients indicated that 55 had normal pressures at rest and during 40 watts of exercise.

The abnormal findings in the remaining 126 patients are summarized in Table 20. The most frequent abnormality, noted in 87 subjects, was an im-

Table 20. Pulmonary hemodynamics (Interpretation of pressure)

	Patients
No examination	19
Normal hemodynamics (rest + exercise)	57
Normal hemodynamics (measured only at rest)	4
Abnormal function during exercise	
Biventricular	87
Left ventricular	22
Right ventricular	10
Abnormal function at rest, insufficiency during exercise	
Biventricular	4
Left ventricular	2
Isolated pulmonary artery hypertension	1
Total	206

Table 21. One-second forced expiratory volume (FEV_1) and bronchial resistance (R) in patients with active pulmonary artery hypertension

No.	Pat.	Age	Sex	PVR[a]	FEV_1 (ml)	FEV_1 (% VC)	R	Operation
1	G.R.	74	M	1.9	1750	55	4.0	Expl. thoracotomy
2	G.E.	63	M	2.0	3200	62	2.3	Lobectomy
3	R.D.	59	M	2.0	2400	76	4.0	Right pneumonectomy
4	C.K.	62	M	2.1	1100	32	9.4	Lobectomy
5	W.H.	62	M	2.2	1800	46	3.6	Bilobectomy
6	W.K.	70	M	2.3	1950	54	4.6	Bilobectomy
7	G.A.	58	M	2.3	1800	50	4.8	Lobectomy
8	H.J.	60	M	2.4	1900	48	4.8	Left pneumonectomy
9	B.K.	59	M	2.7	1600	55	7.7	Lobectomy
10	B.H.	68	M	2.7	1800	54	3.2	Lobectomy
11	M.R.	60	M	2.8	1900	55	4.1	Lobectomy[b]
12	K.K.	56	M	3.2	2250	54	4.6	Left pneumonectomy
13	G.W.	37	M	3.2	1450	42	4.5	Residual pneumonectomy
14	E.J.	50	M	3.3	1050	36	6.6	Lobectomy
15	H.R.	54	M	5.3	1700	48	3.7	Lobectomy

[a] Measured at rest
[b] This patient also underwent a residual pneumonectomy 5½ years later

PVR: Pulmonary vascular resistance ([PAP – LAP]:CO)
R: Bronchial resistance, cm H_2O/L/s

pairment of biventricular function with passive pulmonary artery hypertension during exercise. A passive elevation of pulmonary arterial pressure was also measured in 22 patients who exhibited left ventricular dysfunction during exercise.

Active pulmonary artery hypertension was present in 15 patients, combined in 14 cases with right ventricular or biventricular dysfunction during exercise.

In the absence of congenital or acquired heart disease, active pulmonary artery hypertension is the result of a progressive reduction in the cross-sectional area of the vascular bed of the emphysematous lung [41]. The close relationship between pulmonary obstruction and elevated pulmonary vascular pressure was noted by Herzog in 1966 [129] and by Keller in 1977 [169]. In Table 21 we list the 15 patients diagnosed preoperatively as having active pulmonary artery hypertension in order of increasing measured resistance; measured functional parameters are also shown. The data clearly demonstrate the positive correlation that exists between pulmonary hypertension and impaired lung function. Situations of this kind require particular care in the planning of a pulmonary resection because of the possibility of impaired adaptation of the vascular system.

As the table shows, all but two of the patients (Nos. 2 and 10) had a moderate to severe degree of pulmonary obstruction.

Five patients underwent ventilation and perfusion scanning before surgery was decided upon.

Bronchospirometry and Gaseous Exchange

The degree of function impairment as established by pulmonary function testing and blood gas analyses was assessed semiquantitatively by comparing absolute measured values with tables of normal values and on that basis was categorized as normal, mild, moderate, or severe. Table 22a shows the distribution of restrictive disease, obstructive disease, and their combination. Cases in which these disorders coexisted with diffusion defects are indicated in parentheses.

With 51 patients showing normal pulmonary function and 64 showing mildly impaired function, over half the patients (55%) were identified as good surgical candidates; i.e., they had no significant predictable respiratory problems and were suitable for a pneumonectomy or a lesser resective procedure.

Another 60 patients showed moderate impairments of pulmonary function, over half of which were obstructive. In most cases these disorders were partially reversible by bronchodilation therapy. For patients in this category, partial lung resections carry a slightly increased risk, and pneumonectomies carry a moderate risk.

Twenty-seven other patients had pronounced abnormalities of pulmonary function, most involving a severe obstruction. Even a lobectomy must be considered a high-risk operation in these patients.

To obtain an objective picture of the cases classified as severe, we calculated the mean values of the functional parameters measured in these patients (Table 22b). We were unable to derive useful numerical definitions for the mild

Table 22

a) Impairments of respiratory function

None:	51 patients
Mild:	64 (18)[a] patients
Not measured:	4 patients

Moderate	Type	Severe
38 (9) patients	*Obstruction*	19 (10) patients
12 (4) patients	*Restriction*	3 (–) patients
6 (2) patients	*Combination*	5 (1) patients
4 patients	*Diffusion* (isolated)	–
60 (15) patients	Total	27 (11) patients

b) Mean values of severe respiratory dysfunctions

	Obstruction	Restriction	Combination
TLC	6940 ml (100.5%)	4330 ml (59%)	4840 ml (72.6%)[b]
VC	3390 ml (74.5%)	3000 ml (65%)	2750 ml (58.0%)[b]
FEV_1	1500 ml (44.2%)	2000 ml (66%)	1550 ml (57.0%)[c]
R	6.8	1.9	4.9

[a] Numbers in parentheses indicate patients with coexisting diffusion impairment
[b] Percent predicted value
[c] Percent VC
TLC: Total capacity
VC: Vital capacity
FEV_1: One-second forced expiratory volume
R: Bronchial resistance

and moderate grades of pulmonary dysfunction, as Geddes et al. [91] were able to do in their prospective study.

It must be emphasized that especially the obstructive forms of respiratory dysfunction can be positively influenced by preoperative measures such as cessation of smoking, antibronchitic therapy, and respiratory exercises [267, 361]. Perruchoud et al. [264] showed that when these measures are implemented, many patients previously classified as "inoperable" become acceptable surgical candidates.

The Effects of Thoracic Surgical Procedures on Pulmonary Function and Hemodynamics

The acceptance of pulmonary functional status as a risk factor emphasizes the importance of knowing the changes that result from thoracotomy and the resection of lung parenchyma. This question has been the subject of numerous studies.

Respiratory Consequences

A comprehensive account of the pathophysiologic sequelae of major thoracic surgery is found in Schilling [290]. Thoracotomy in itself, without lung resection, can temporarily decrease vital capacity by up to 50% of the initial value. This is the expression of a restrictive condition which, in the absence of complications, rarely persists longer than 2–3 weeks.

Studies by Harms et al. [114] demonstrate the presence of alveolar hypoventilation with arterial hypoxemia and hypercapnia in the early postoperative period after partial lung resections. The severity of this condition increases until the second postoperative day.

Nolte [243] compared preoperative vital capacity with that measured 1–3 weeks after exploratory thoracotomy, pneumonectomy, and lobectomy and found average reductions of 25%, 40%, and 45%, respectively. The greater reduction after lobectomy compared with pneumonectomy may seem surprising at first but is explained by cases where pneumonectomy was performed on a lung that had already lost much of its function prior to operation.

Berend et al. [26] monitored respiration and ventilation for periods of 6 weeks to 6 months after lobectomies. They found that the vital capacity and one-second forced expiratory volume were reduced by only 12%. Navratil et al. [238] performed spirometric tests at 6-month intervals for 3 years following lobectomy and pneumonectomy. The average reduction of VC and FEV_1 after lobectomy was 15% and 20%, respectively. The FEV_1 declined even further with passage of time. As expected, pneumonectomy resulted in more substantial losses, specifically a 30%–40% reduction of VC and FEV_1. By the end of the 3-year study the postpneumonectomy FEV_1 had fallen an average of 45% relative to the preoperative value. According to investigations by Jones et al. [160], the VC was still 50% of the normal value 10–15 years after pneumonectomy. Blood gas analyses indicated no adverse changes following either type of resection [34, 220, 226, 233].

Veneskoski et al. [343a] examined 39 patients who had undergone lobectomies, 19 of whom were carcinoma patients. They found an initial VC reduction of approximately 12% in the carcinoma group and an approximately 20% reduction of FEV_1. Twelve months after surgery there was still an approximately 9% loss of vital capacity, while the FEV_1 remained about 15% below the preoperative value. These values are more favorable than those reported by Navratil.

Laros [186a] published lung function data on 123 patients who were followed for 20 years after total pneumonectomy. Most of these were tuberculosis patients who had undergone surgery at a relatively young age. The data indicate an approximately 40-ml loss of vital capacity per decade of life, as opposed to an average of 100–380 ml in age-matched controls. Of course, one must be careful about applying these results to the considerably older population of carcinoma patients, who have a higher prevalence of associated obstructive bronchitis.

In summary, it may be said that thoracic surgical operations lead in the early phase to disturbances of diffusion and ventilation and to a predominantly restrictive volume loss. Abnormalities of diffusion and ventilation are the most easily reversible. Restriction of ventilation, which is reinforced by postoperative pain, is maximal in the first two weeks after surgery. Later it is proportional to the extent of the resection. This pattern is not characteristic in cases where the resected lung segment was nonfunctional or partially nonfunctional prior to surgery.

Effect on Pulmonary Hemodynamics

Every lung resection results in reduction of the pulmonary vascular bed. In theory, this leads to an increase in pulmonary vascular resistance and places an increased pressure load on the right ventricle. Daum et al. [60] showed that unilateral occlusion of the pulmonary artery in healthy subjects does not raise the *mean arterial pressure* at rest, and that during exercise (50–70 watts) it raises it less than 4 mm Hg relative to the pressure during bilateral perfusion. Brofman et al. [41] measured the *pulmonary systolic pressure* in 8 healthy subjects and found an average increase of 50% following unilateral pulmonary artery occlusion.

Stanek et al. [326] measured pulmonary artery pressure in patients who had undergone pneumonectomy. In the patients less than 50 years of age, the mean arterial pressure was 18 mm Hg at rest and 28 mm Hg during exercise – values that are just within upper normal limits (Daum et al. [60]). In older patients, who had a slightly elevated initial value (PAP_{mean} = 21 mm Hg), the pressure rose to 40 mm Hg during exercise.

Pulmonary artery pressure measurements made by Johansson et al. [157] during the first 2 days after pneumonectomy, lobectomy, or thoracotomy without resection showed no significant differences between these groups other than a slight fall of cardiac output in the pneumonectomized patients.

Perceptions Regarding Functional Tolerance Limits

Concepts concerning the operability of lung cancer patients are based in large part on empirical observations relating to operative mortality, the incidence of postoperative complications, and long-term morbidity from cardiorespiratory insufficiency.

Hartel et al. [115], in a 1969 study involving intraoperative measurements of pulmonary arterial pressure, made the clinically important observation that pneumonectomized patients in particular have a markedly reduced tolerance toward rapid fluid administration.

Pecora and Brook [263] analyzed 12 deaths among 176 patients who underwent lung resections (= 7%). They found a correlation between the mean pulmonary artery pressure (measured intraoperatively) and the operative mortality, which was 3.2% at pressures to 26 mm Hg, 20% at pressures to 30 mm Hg, and 66% at pressures over 30 mm Hg. (Pressures are converted from cm H_2O to mm Hg.) It must be added that these pressures were measured under conditions of general anesthesia and controlled ventilation and therefore should be interpreted only in relative terms.

Daum et al. [60] discovered that all 8 of 30 pneumonectomized patients who died within one year after surgery had a preoperative mean pulmonary artery pressure greater than 28 mm Hg at rest. Right heart failure was confirmed in three of these patients.

Schickedanz and Voelkner [289] performed right heart catheterization in 263 patients prior to lung resection. Thirty-three of these patients (12.5%) did not survive the operation. The mean pulmonary *systolic* pressure in the group of nonsurvivors was 32 mm Hg – 30% higher than in the survivors. It is not stated whether the measurements were performed at rest or during exercise, although the former may be presumed. The authors conclude that the 33 deaths were the result of right heart failure, without citing specific evidence to support their conclusion.

It has been suggested that the response of the pulmonary artery pressure to lung resection, especially pneumonectomy, be predicted by measuring pressure while a balloon catheter occludes the side requiring operation [60]. Elevations of the mean artery pressure by more than 7 mm Hg, and the occurrence of arterial hypoxemia and hypercapnia, are considered an unfavorable prognostic sign and a contraindication to pneumonectomy. Olsen et al. [248] and Freisleben [87] state that a mean pulmonary artery pressure of more than 35 mm Hg during exercise is a contraindication – a value that is consistent with our guidelines.

Chapter 4

Operative Treatment

History

The first successful resection of a lung carcinoma was performed by the American surgeon E. A. Graham in St. Louis in 1933 [351]. His patient, a 48-year-old physician, was able to resume his medical practice and lived until 1964 without experiencing a recurrence. Graham resected the involved lung, implanted radium seeds in the bronchial stump for suspected hilar node metastases, and also performed a thoracoplasty, removing seven ribs. With the former measure he apparently provoked the stump insufficiency that ensued, and with the latter he prevented its potentially fatal consequences.

Since the spectacular success of this pioneering operation, there has been a trend toward the systematization of resective therapy. In 1948 Brock [37] stated that the only adequate tumor resection was a pneumonectomy, and that a "radical" pneumonectomy with intrapericardial division of the major pulmonary vessels and excision of the regional lymph nodes (a "block-dissection" pneumonectomy) was the best technique. In the decades that followed, however, lobectomy came to be regarded as an acceptable form of treatment in some instances, and some authors [155, 317, 335, 364] even advocated a segmental resection or local wedge resection in selected cases. It is apparent that a limited resection extends the potential benefits of surgical treatment to patients who would be unable to tolerate a pneumonectomy, and that the immediate operative risk and long-term function impairment are less than with the more extensive operation. Today there is little question that lobectomy offers cure rates and survival rates in early-stage cancer patients that are comparable to those obtained with pneumonectomy.

Definition of Terms

A major difficulty in interpreting the results of surgical treatment lies in the ambiguous use of operative terms [27]. As early as 1960, Lawrence et al. [190] pointed to the need for a standardized terminology.

This problem is illustrated by the different uses of the word "radical." Since the works of Brock [38], Brock and Whytehead [40], and Cahen [46], "radical" is used in the American and British literature to describe a pneumonectomy (Brock) or lobectomy (Cahen) combined with en bloc resection of the mediastinal fat and lymph nodes. The term is similarly applied to a mastectomy that involves en bloc removal of the axillary lymph nodes. But in the surgery of lung carcinoma, it is very common for authors to use "radical" as a synonym for "complete." Sommerwerck [317] speaks of "radical" operations in connection with parenchyma-conserving wedge resections and defends this usage on etymologic grounds. Zeidler [369] considers the English term "radical resection" to be somewhat vague and quotes the American authors Ramsey et al. [273], who used "radical" in the sense of "standard." However, these authors correctly draw a distinction between "simple" and "radical" as an operative principle. This distinction is maintained by the British authors Robinson and Burkell [276]. Yet even in recent publications, one still finds confusing terms such as "simple radical pneumonectomy" [92] and "extended radical operation".

The confusion becomes even greater when the term "palliative" is used as the opposite of "radical" (e.g., [92, 94]) in the sense of "incomplete." An incomplete resection may indeed be done for the purpose of palliation, but the term "palliative" describes the preoperative or intraoperative election of a therapy whose intent is not a definitive cure, but the immediate relief of suffering or improvement of the quality of life. An example would be a complete local tumor resection in the presence of distant metastases. Accordingly, when the decision is made to undertake a palliative operation, the usual oncologic criteria of resectability no longer apply, or else the procedure is performed without bothering to evaluate the patient for possible contraindications.

Similar misunderstandings arise in connection with the term "extended resection." Its correct definition is the resection of extrapulmonary structures that have been invaded by lung tumor (Kutschera, 1971 [181, 184]). Hence, the basic prerequisite for an extended resection is the presence of a T3 neoplasm. Kutschera, while formulating his definition, reports on extended resections in stage II cases. If we follow his discussion, we find that lobectomies which include a sleeve of the main bronchus serving the resected lobe (cf. p. 58) are counted as extended resections, as is the intrapericardial ligation and division of the hilar vessels, which may be necessary for technical reasons even when the pericardium is not involved by tumor. Zeidler [369] also regards the sleeve lobectomy as a type of extended resection. Many such examples could be cited.

So that the procedures analyzed in our study may be classified without ambiguity, and to provide a basis for discussion and possibly for a generally valid nomenclature, we propose the following terms that relate to three different aspects of resective lung surgery:

a) Type of Procedure

Simple or *standard* lobectomy/pneumonectomy

A resection that does not involve systematic dissection of the regional lymph nodes. This does not pertain to the random removal of lymph nodes for intraoperative staging.

Radical lobectomy/pneumonectomy
En bloc resection of the lung or a pulmonary lobe with concomitant removal of the ipsilateral mediastinal lymphatic system. For technical reasons this generally includes (in pneumonectomies) the intrapericardial division of the major pulmonary vessels.

Sleeve lobectomy
Technical alternative to pneumonectomy for tumors that cannot be removed with an adequate safety margin simply by dividing the bronchus at its junction with the more proximal bronchial segment. This procedure is used when the risk of pneumonectomy appears to be prohibitive for functional reasons.

Extended lobectomy/pneumonectomy
This refers to the resection of the tumor-bearing segment, lobe, or lung together with adjacent structures that are invaded by tumor. Examples are pneumonectomy combined with resection of the pericardium and/or atrium for a centrally located tumor, and lobectomy or pneumonectomy combined with resection of chest wall or the diaphragm for a peripheral tumor. This category includes resections that must be extended to the trachea.

b) Gross and Histologic Adequacy of Local Resection

Complete resection
Resection that includes a tissue margin that is free of tumor according to gross assessment and histologic testing. The central lymph nodes (hilar in a pneumonectomy, interlobar in a lobectomy) must be free of tumor.

Questionably complete resection
The safety margin between the line of resection and tumor is less than 2 cm. There is intranodal tumor growth in adjacent lymph nodes.

Incomplete resection
The line of resection passes grossly *through* the tumor, or histologic examination shows tumor extending to the resected margin (submucous or peribronchial, in cancellous bone of rib with chest wall infiltration, etc.).

An incomplete resection can usually be avoided by using intraoperative frozen-section examinations to confirm the adequacy of the resection and show whether additional pulmonary tissue should be resected.

c) Prognostic Assessment of Surgical Treatment

Curative resection
Locally complete resection of T1 or T2 lesion in the absence of distant and mediastinal metastases.

Questionably curative resection
Complete, extended resection of a T3 lesion and/or radical resection for ipsilateral lymph node involvement (N2).

Noncurative resection
All locally incomplete resections, or all locally complete resections associated with known hematogenous and/or inaccessible lymphatic metastases.

These terms are similar to those that were coined in 1959 by Chamberlain et al. [51] and were adopted and expanded by R. A. Smith [313, 314]. They are sufficient to provide an unambiguous description of a resective lung operation.

These terms are to be distinguished from terms that characterize indications. The preferred and by far the most common indication is for curative resection. Accordingly, the list of contraindications includes findings which make a curative resection questionable, unlikely, or impossible (cf. p. 67).

When the indication for surgery is palliative, the resection is performed not with the intent to cure, but to make the patient more comfortable in the short term. A palliative resection may be elected preoperatively or, intraoperatively, as an alternative to exploratory thoracotomy. When elected preoperatively, the palliative resection usually aims at relieving intolerable symptoms even if the presence of distant metastases is known or suspected.

A third possibility is that the resection is performed as an *adjuvant* procedure. This refers to the resection of a lung tumor that is not causing local symptoms despite known distant metastasis. It is likely that adjuvant resections will gain increasing importance as part of an interdisciplinary program of treatment.

Applied Principles

Consistent principles were applied to the selection of surgical procedures in the series. These principles agree with the consensus of surgical opinion as expressed in the literature [152, 153], with a basic distinction made between operations with curative intent and palliative procedures.

Unlike some authors [43, 180, 317, 364], we reject segmental and wedge resections as curative operations for primary lung carcinoma. If the cardiorespiratory function of a patient is so severely compromised that he would be unable to tolerate the loss of a lobe, then the function impairment caused by thoracotomy alone would be sufficient to create an unacceptable risk in the early postoperative period (cf. p. 50). Accordingly, we feel that the procedures of lobectomy, right bilobectomy, and pneumonectomy are most appropriate to the goal of complete eradication in lung carcinoma. The present series includes only one patient who underwent a wedge resection for a lesion presumed to be metastatic from an extrapulmonary adenocarcinoma. Twenty-one months later this assessment was proved incorrect by autopsy findings.

Both the stage and the location of the tumor have an important bearing on the necessary extent of the resection. Stage I disease often can be managed by lobectomy, although a pneumonectomy may prove necessary for a small carcinoma that has reached a lobar bronchus (Fig. 11). With stage II cancer, which features limited lymph node involvement (N 1), pneumonectomy is the operation of choice provided the condition can be diagnosed before or during surgery (positive interlobar or hilar lymph nodes). A possible alternative is the radical lobectomy described by Cahen, although the authors (Cahen [46] and

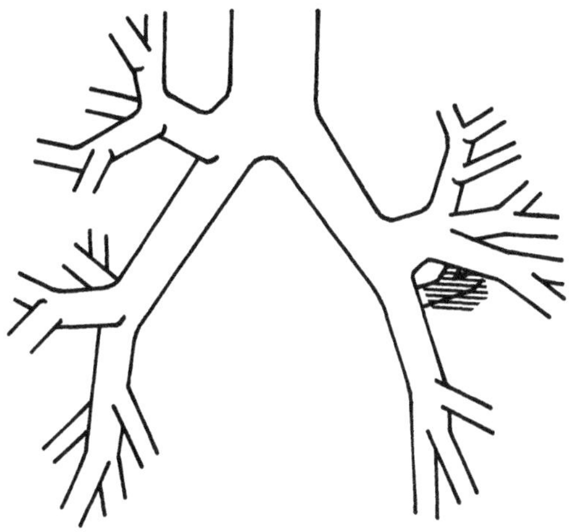

Fig. 11. Schematic drawing of a carcinoma in the S6 left segmental bronchus. A tumor less than 3 cm in diameter satisfies the criteria of a T_1 lesion. Because of its proximity to the upper lobar orifice, however, a pneumonectomy is often indicated

Ramsey et al. [273]) themselves caution that this procedure does not always achieve the completeness of a pneumonectomy. In any case, many patients are not identified as stage II cases until after surgery, when histopathologic examination of the surgical specimen reveals metastases in intralobar lymph nodes. If extrapulmonary lymph nodes are known to be involved by tumor, one must undertake a more extensive operation that includes lymphadenectomy (radical pneumonectomy of Brock). If there is infiltration of extrapulmonary structures, an extended resection will be required. The factors that determine the approach that is most suitable for a particular patient are:

a) preoperative findings, including bronchoscopic findings noted by the surgeon himself;
b) inspection and palpation in the thoracotomized chest;
c) liberal use of frozen-section examinations, especially of lymph node specimens taken at operation.

Simple Lobectomy

The resection of a single pulmonary lobe can be curative for many carcinomas of the T1 and T2 categories. However, an endobronchial tumor that extends farther centrally than the origin of a segmental bronchus is not curable by a usual lobectomy, because there is not adequate clearance between the tumor margin and the line of resection.

Certain carcinomas that grow within or compress a lobar bronchus (T2) can be removed either by the "sleeve" technique or with a bilobectomy. In the first case the resection is extended to the mainstem bronchus, followed by a bronchial anastomosis; in the second case the resection includes the adjacent lobe, such that the line of bronchial resection passes through the right mainstem bronchus.

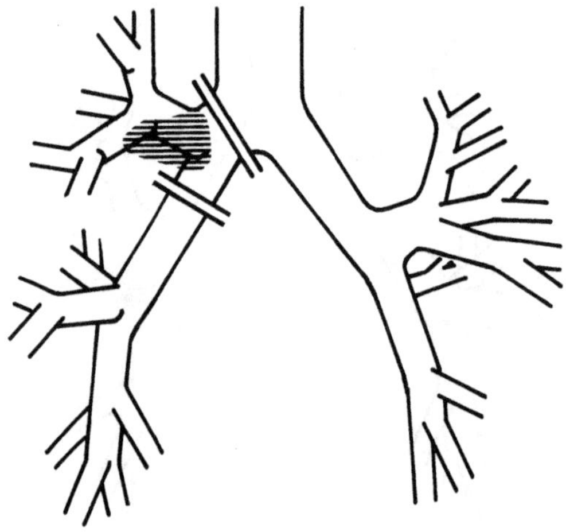

Fig. 12. Principle of the sleeve resection with subsequent bronchial anastomosis. The "classic" indication is carcinoma involving the upper lobar orifice of the right lung

Sleeve Lobectomy (Fig. 12)

The sleeve lobectomy is a special procedure that is used when a simple lobectomy cannot provide complete removal of the tumor, yet a pneumonectomy is contraindicated on functional grounds.

The tumor-bearing lobe is resected together with a segment of the main bronchus. Continuity is restored with an end-to-end anastomosis. For anatomic reasons this procedure is most appropriate for carcinomas occurring at the inlet of the right upper lobar bronchus [237, 256, 269, 271]. Otherwise such tumors are removable only by pneumonectomy, even if their local extent is small.

The present series includes seven upper lobectomies, five on the right side and two on the left, that were performed using the sleeve technique. This corresponds to 6% of all lobectomies or 4% of all resections.

Larger numbers are reported by Thompson [333], Naef [234–236], Paneth [251], Shaw and Luke [300], and Jensik [155]. McHale [204] and Thompson [333] favor the sleeve technique when there is invasion of the pulmonary artery, in which case a vascular anastomosis also must be performed.

All authors state that the complication rate and operative mortality are lower than in pneumonectomies and marginally higher than in simple lobectomies.

Given the small number of sleeve lobectomies in our series, the one postoperative death must be regarded as significant, although local complications did not contribute to the fatal outcome. We encountered no instances of anastomotic insufficiency. Retained secretions in four patients, necessitating one or more endoscopic aspirations, are virtually pathognomonic for sleeve resections [154, 256, 320].

A more serious problem, we feel, is the relative inability of the sleeve resection to eradicate lymph node metastases compared with pneumonectomy, even when the tumor is excised with an adequate margin of healthy tissue. Certainly, the dissection of involved interlobar lymph nodes is less curative than when a total pneumonectomy is performed.

Table 23. Sleeve lobectomies (All for squamous cell carcinoma)

Patient	TNM	Resection	Course
H.H., 73	T2, N1, M0	Left upper lobe	Died 38 months postop. with generalized metastases
S.F., 63	T2, N1, M0	Left upper lobe	Died 9 months postop. with local re-recurrence and generalized spread
B.J., 65	T2, N1, M0	Right upper lobe	Died 14 months postop. with clinical evidence of local recurrence
G.K., 66	T2, N0, M0	Right upper lobe	Died 5 weeks postop. from cerebral insult
B.K., 59	T2, N0, M0	Right upper lobe	Died 16 months postop. with no clinical evidence of recurrence; autopsy was not performed
T.P., 63	T2, N0, M0	Right upper lobe	Died 5 months postop. with urothelial carcinoma; autopsy showed no recurrence
H.E., 73	T2, N0, M0	Right upper lobe	Died 5 years postop. with squamous carcinoma of the left side

In three patients with squamous cell carcinoma, metastatic tumor was present in intra- and interlobar nodes, but the patients were not considered acceptable candidates for pneumonectomy. Two of these patients died 9 months and 14 months after operation with clinical or autopsy evidence of local recurrence.

Of the remaining 3 patients, 1 died 5 years postoperatively from a carcinoma of the contralateral side, 1 patient (not autopsied) died after 16 months with no clinical evidence of tumor progression, and 1 died 5 months postoperatively from a urothelial carcinoma (Table 23).

Bilobectomy (Fig. 13)

Bilobectomy is a partial resection performed on the trilobate right lung. A lower bilobectomy, with resection of the middle and inferior lobes, is the more common type and is performed for tumor growth involving the middle lobar bronchus or the inlet of the inferior lobe. The less common upper bilobectomy is indicated for peripheral carcinomas that exhibit translobar growth. Not infrequently, a congenitally deficient pulmonary fissure is responsible for this pattern of tumor growth.

We applied strict criteria to the utilization of the special lobectomies described above. If a patient's preoperative functional status was good, pneumonectomy was considered the procedure of choice.

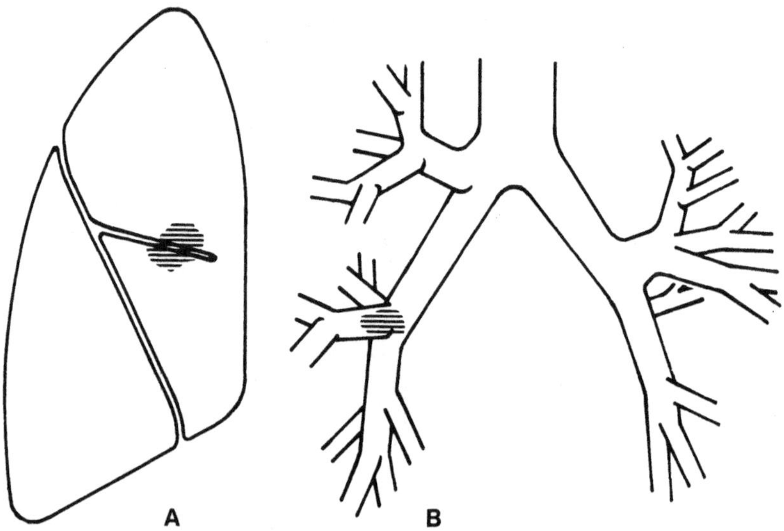

Fig. 13 A, B. Indications for bilobectomy of the right lung. **A** Peripheral translobar tumor (upper bilobectomy). **B** Endobronchial tumor involving the middle lobar orifice or distal mainstem bronchus (lower bilobectomy)

Simple Pneumonectomy

While some authors routinely favor en bloc resection of the lung and mediastinal nodes according to the method of Brock, we perform a simple resection when no evidence of hilar or mediastinal metastasis is apparent at mediastinoscopy or at operation.

Pneumonectomy is indicated for all peripheral, translobar tumors of the left lung and in all cases where endobronchial tumor growth involves a lobar bronchus. In selected cases a right pneumonectomy may be avoided in favor of a lesser operation, as stated above.

Radical Pneumonectomy

A radical pneumonectomy is indicated whenever the hilar and mediastinal lymph nodes are involved by tumor. Thus, the N status of a case dictates the necessity of this operation. If N 2 involvement is detected by preoperative mediastinoscopy, the radical technique is incorporated into the plan of operation; if the metastasis is discovered at operation, the technique is selected ad hoc. N 2 lesions are potentially curable by surgery alone, but the outcome is questionable. Surgery should be followed whenever possible by irradiation of the mediastinum and supraclavicular fields (see pp. 91).

Radical Lobectomy

We do not employ radical lobectomy as a standard procedure, because it is questionable whether dissection of the interlobar lymph nodes and subsequent removal of the hilar and mediastinal nodes can guarantee a complete eradication of disease. This is because the peribronchial lymphatics remain intact in the area of the bronchial stump and along the mainstem bronchus, and they may provide a reservoir for malignant cells. We reserve radical lobectomy for patients who are functionally unable to tolerate a pneumonectomy.

Extended Pneumonectomy

In some cases extended pneumonectomies are planned procedures that are elected when preoperative tests show endobronchial tumor growth in proximity to the carina, phrenic nerve paralysis points to invasion of the pericardium anterior to the lung root, or there is circumscribed chest wall invasion with no evidence of diffuse pleural involvement or effusion. More frequently, however, the need for an extended pneumonectomy is not apparent until a T3 lesion is discovered at operation. The histology of the neoplasm, the condition and age of the patient, and the likelihood of tumor-related complications will dictate whether it is better to perform an extended resection or terminate the procedure as an exploratory thoracotomy. The success of an extended pneumonectomy is at best questionable. Some of these resections are not complete, and most are combined with adjuvant postoperative radiotherapy.

Extended Lobectomy

This procedure is analogous to the extended pneumonectomy, i.e., the lobe is resected together with involved adjacent structures. Almost invariably, the resection is extended to portions of the chest wall or diaphragm (Fig. 14) that have been directly invaded by a peripheral carcinoma.

A special case is represented by "Pancoast's tumor," or superior sulcus carcinoma (Pancoast [250]). This term is applied to tumors, mostly squamous cell carcinomas and undifferentiated large cell carcinomas, that arise from the apex of the lung, penetrate the thoracic inlet, and produce characteristic symptoms. The cardinal symptoms are neurologic deficits and pain in the region of the brachiocervical plexus and, with involvement of the sympathetic trunk, Horner's syndrome. The accepted treatment for these tumors is preliminary radiotherapy followed by an extended lobectomy with rib and plexus resection [19]. Paulson and Urschel [255] report a 5-year survival rate of approximately 30%. A more recent publication by Paulson [253a] dealing with 68 cases managed by combined radiotherapy and extended resection reports a 5-year survival of almost 35%, with a greater than 44% survival in the absence of lymph node metastases. A substantial number of patients have attained 10 or even 15 years of sur-

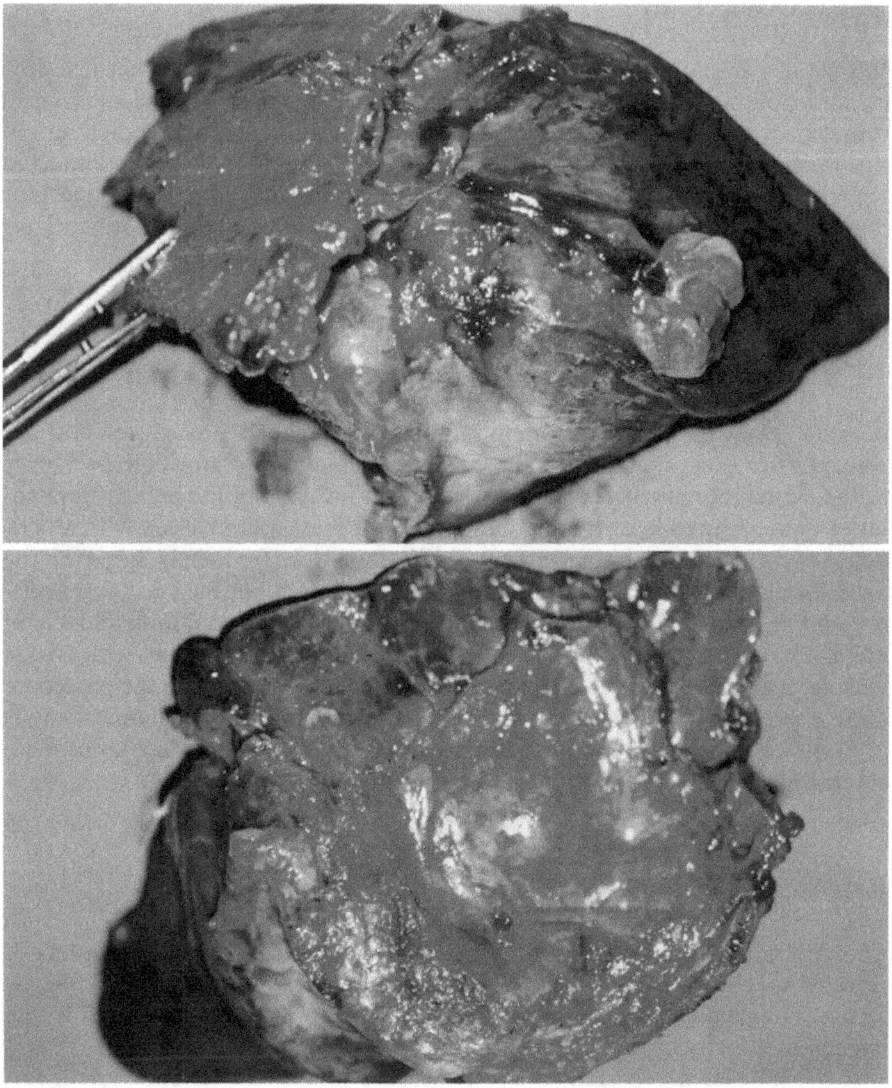

Fig. 14. Surgical specimen from an extended left lower lobectomy for squamous cell carcinoma. *Top:* View of three rib cross-sections (left in photo). *Bottom:* View of the peritoneal surface of the diaphragm with central tumor bulge

vival. Only 2 operative deaths are reported in a total of 68 resections (2.9%). It should be emphasized, however, that the alleviation of pain in itself is sufficient indication for resective surgery. Like the pneumonectomies, we consider extended lobectomies to be questionably curative at best.

Characteristics of the Resections

Overview

The resections performed in the present series can be grouped into categories in accordance with the above guidelines for adequate resection techniques and our definitions of the terms "radical" and "extended" (Table 24).

One hundred thirty-nine of the resections were simple lobectomies or simple pneumonectomies. Being potentially curative, these procedures were not supplemented by adjuvant measures. In 24 cases we performed concomitant regional lymph node dissections, most of which were done in conjunction with pneumonectomies. Twenty-nine patients underwent extended resections, again mostly in pneumonectomies. It should be noted that extended resection does not preclude lymphadenectomy and is frequently combined with it.

Palliative Resections

In seven cases the primary indication for surgery was palliative. Six of these patients did not undergo mediastinoscopy before surgery. One patient had refused invasive testing 16 months previously and another had refused resective therapy 6 months previously, leading in each case to advanced disease and significant tumor-related complications. A grossly and histologically complete resection was accomplished in four patients. In two patients the resection was incomplete; in another the lesion was technically nonresectable (Table 25).

In contrast to the primary palliative operations in which half of the local resections were complete, the secondary palliative operations were by definition incomplete. It was decided intraoperatively to remove the tumor-bearing lobe,

Table 24. Overview of the technical aspects of resections

	n	%
A. Pneumonectomies		
1. Simple	42	59
2. Radical	11	15
3. Extended	18	26
Total	71	100
B. Lobectomies (incl. sleeve and bilob.)		
1. Simple	97	80
2. Radical	13	11
3. Extended	11	9
Total	121	100

Table 25. Primary palliative operations

Pat.	Age	Histol.	Reason for palliation	Operation	Length of survival
F.N.	74	Squam	Fetid sputum, radiol. necrosis	Bilobectomy, complete	19 months[a]
S.A.	65	Squam	Fetid sputum, fever, radiol. necrosis	Lobectomy, complete	20 months[a]
H.R.	54	LCC	Pain, radiol. rib destruction	Lobectomy, chest wall resection, incomplete, pos. cytology, pleural effusion	2 months[a]
S.P.	68	Squam	Fetid sputum, rib metastases	Pneumonectomy, incomplete (ribs, LN metastases)	6 months[a]
E.H.	58	LCC	Severe hemoptysis (emergency op.)	Pneumonectomy, complete	6 years[b]
B.C.	62	SCC	Inflow statis, extreme dyspnea, no histology	Venoatrial shunt	16 months[a]

[a] Cause of death: Tumor progression
[b] Incurrent surgery and radiotherapy for brain metastases
Squam: Squamous cell carcinoma
LCC: Large cell undifferentiated carcinoma
SCC: Small cell carcinoma

leaving behind residual tumor in the mediastinum or chest wall. One patient even required a pneumonectomy. Most cases involved the palliative removal of necrotic tumor masses, which were considered to preclude a simple exploratory procedure. The operation gave three patients a longer symptom-free survival despite the fact that tumor was left behind. One patient died postoperatively (Table 26).

Adjuvant Resections

Adjuvant resections were performed in two young patients with adenocarcinoma. In both cases evaluation was delayed through the fault of the attending physician. Both cases were judged a priori to be surgically incurable, but there was no indication for the alleviation of an acutely threatening condition. Rather, resection of the primary tumor was intended as part of an interdisciplinary treatment program.

1) Patient B. T., f., 44 years of age (Fig. 10). A chest X-ray taken in March, 1968, showed a small density in the left lower lung. The next X-ray taken in July, 1973, when the patient was asymptomatic showed a 7-cm round shadow in the left supradiaphragmatic area diagnosed as tuberculosis. At hospitalization 4½ months later routine preoperative cancer tests were negative until mediastinoscopy showed bilateral metastatic involvement of

Table 26. Secondary (intraoperative) palliative operations

Pat.	Age	Histol.	Reason for palliation	Operation	Length of survival
B.H.	61	Squam	Invasion of chest wall and vertebrae	Bilobectomy	7 months
K.H.	48	Adeno	Invasion of aortic arch	Lobectomy, LN dissection, incomplete	Op. death
M.E.	72	Squam	Penetration of chest wall	Lobectomy, chest wall, incomplete	6 months
M.H.	60	Adeno	Penetration of mediastinum, tumor necrosis + +, metastasis in same lobe	Lobectomy, incomplete	31 months
M.W.	51	Squam	Direct pretracheal invasion	Lobectomy, incomplete	16 months
R.E.	72	LCC	Tumor abscess, pleural invasion at thoracic apex (Fig. 15)	Lobectomy, incomplete	24 months
R.M.	56	LCC	Invasion of chest wall	Bilobectomy, chest wall, incomplete	9 months
B.A.	73	Squam	Wide necrotic invasion of mediastinum	Pneumonectomy, extended, incomplete	4 months

Squam: Squamous cell carcinoma
Adeno: Adenocarcinoma
LCC: Large cell undifferentiated carcinoma

nonenlarged paratracheal, tracheobronchial, and subcarinal nodes. The tumor was removed by lobectomy.

The mediastinum was irradiated with a curative dose of 6000 rads. Clinical examination at 6 months showed bilateral pleuritis and pericarditis. After 18 months neurologic symptoms were noted, and CT scans showed multiple brain metastases. The patient died 24 months postoperatively. Autopsy was not performed.

2) Patient W. U., m., 34 years of age. Slight hemoptysis noted in September, 1974, was treated as catharrh. Hemoptysis recurred in December (3 times), and a course of antibiotics was prescribed. A chest X-ray taken in April, 1975, as part of a sport fitness examination (diving) showed infiltrate in the left lower lung. This was accompanied by the complaint of paresthesia in the left little finger. Four weeks later the patient presented with high fever, and X-ray showed marked enlargement of the infiltrate. Patient was hospitalized in June, 1975. Sputum cytology indicated an undifferentiated tumor. CT scans showed brain metastases in the right temportal area.

Brain irradiation was initiated. Adjuvant resection was scheduled without evidence of other distant metastasis and without mediastinoscopy. The primary tumor (5-cm adenocarcinoma) was completely removed by lobectomy combined with dissection of metastatically involved interlobar and hilar nodes. Cytostatic therapy followed.

Bone metastases were detected 12 months after surgery, prompting radiotherapy of the spine and pelvis for pain relief. Patient died 16 months postoperatively. Autopsy showed metastases in the brain, liver, skeleton, abdominal and thoracic lymph nodes, and pleura, and carcinomatous lymphangitis in both lungs.

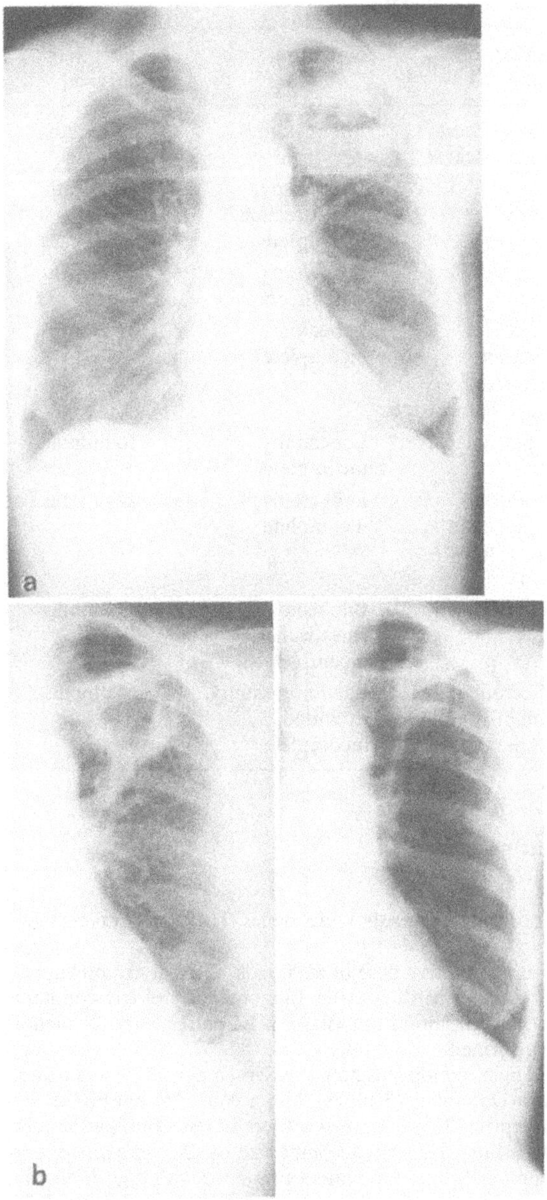

Fig. 15. a Example of a situation warranting secondary (intraoperative) palliation. The radiograph shows a tumor cavity with a fluid level in the left upper lung (cT2). Apical chest wall invasion was found at operation, indicating a pT3 lesion (cf. Fig. 6). An incomplete resection was performed, and the patient survived 24 months (R. E., f., 72 years of age, PA chest film). **b** Radiograph of same patient showing the appearance of the left upper lobe 8 months (*left*) and 5 months (*right*) before resection. The diagnosis of malignancy was missed because of negative cytology and a reduction of tumor size during antibiotic therapy

The impact of these operations on survival time is difficult to assess with any accuracy. Nevertheless, it is clear that rapid tumor growth probably would have caused pulmonary complications if resection had not been carried out.

Another adjuvant resection was done in a 54-year-old man with an unclassified lung carcinoma of the right apex and Pancoast-like symptoms. The diagnosis of malignancy was made five months after the onset of unexplained pain and progressive weakness in the right arm. Following the recommendations of Becker et al. [19], the lesion was first irradiated at a dose of 6000 rads. This was followed by surgical extirpation with an extended upper lobectomy. Three months later brain metastases were diagnosed. Despite partial resection of the metastases and brain irradiation, the patient died from cancer cachexia eight months after pulmonary resection.

Oncologic Contraindications

Opinions on when the resection of a lung carcinoma is still appropriate and when surgical treatment should no longer be considered vary from one center to the next and over the course of time. Fifteen or 20 years ago this question was still being addressed in the majority of surgical studies. With the general trend toward a more aggressive therapeutic approach, relatively little attention is given to this problem in the recent literature. Today it is more common to discuss the forms of mediastinal lymph node involvement that may be amenable to surgery. In recent years there has been reexamination of the question of whether surgery has a role in the treatment of small cell carcinoma, although for years it was widely held that this type of cancer categorically precludes surgery. Indeed, when a consistent system is utilized for the classification and staging of tumors, the only contraindications that must be considered pertain to cases of stage III disease. By definition, it is agreed that patients with non-small cell carcinoma of clinical stage I or II are acceptable surgical candidates from an oncologic standpoint.

In the present series the following criteria for nonoperability were used throughout the period of the study (and also at the present time):

Absolute contraindications
Distant metastasis
Contralateral lymph node metastasis
Upper inflow stasis
Recurrent laryngeal nerve paralysis
Invasion of the trachea
Invasion of the esophagus
Invasion of the chest wall outside the costal thorax
Pleural effusion with malignant cells

Relative contraindications
Ipsilateral lymph node metastasis by undifferentiated carcinoma
Ipsilateral lymph node metastasis with penetration of the capsule
Phrenic nerve paralysis with a peripherally located tumor

This list of findings that preclude surgical resection agrees basically with the criteria of Belcher and Anderson [21], Matthes [209], Robinson and Burkell [276], Salzer [288], Rossetti [279], and Mittman and Bruderman [224].

Tumor invasion of the thoracic apex (superior sulcus tumor, Pancoast's tumor) was identified in 1970 by Salzer and by Robinson and Burkell as a contraindication to surgery. Sensenig et al. [297] stated that any chest wall invasion should preclude resection, while Kraft-Kinz et al. [175] cited phrenic nerve paralysis as an absolute contraindication. Schoen and Stoehr [291] "usually" rejected surgery for any form of mediastinal lymph node metastasis.

Other authors [3, 83, 186, 283, 370] regard ipsilateral metastasis as a criterion for nonoperability only if the patient is elderly or in poor health, or in cases of poorly differentiated tumor.

The list of contraindications presented by Zwintz [371] is considerably less restrictive. Operable solitary distant metastases of the brain and bone do not preclude resection in every case. Local invasion of the trachea, aorta, esophagus, spine, or vena cava is prohibitive only if it is circumferential or too extensive (e.g., with penetration of the spinal canal).

As the list of contraindications is shortened, the readiness to perform extended resections must increase accordingly.

For example, MacHale [204], in 1972, described a method for excision of the tracheal bifurcation followed by bronchoplastic repair. Additional bronchoplastic procedures for various tumor locations are described by Naruke et al. [237] and Zeidler [369]. Techniques are also available for prosthetic vascular replacement and for repairing and stabilizing chest wall defects with alloplastic material. In a report on 43 resections of bronchial carcinoma invading the chest wall, Jamieson et al. [151] state a primary mortality of 16%. Three patients survived for three years, and three others survived for five years, corresponding to a long-term success rate of less than 14%.

In selected cases of this series we disregarded our standard list of contraindications, electing in a few instances to perform surgery in the face of bilateral lymph node involvement or known distant metastases. It should be emphasized that our own experiences and those related in the literature do not justify a basically more liberal approach to the use of surgical resection in all lung cancer patients. However, when the chest is open and the surgeon is confronted with unexpectedly advanced disease, it is easier to justify the decision to extend the procedure even if it conflicts with established rules.

Postoperative Complications

As our review of the results of the function tests indicates, a great many patients suffered not only from their lung cancer but also from disturbances of cardiorespiratory function not causally related to the tumor. Operations on an organ system with preexisting disease whose function is quantitatively impaired pose a considerable risk of decompensation and can lead to potentially serious problems in the postoperative period. Given the advanced age of most lung cancer patients, latent or overt disorders of other organ systems can become significant in connection with the stress of anesthesia and surgery.

As popularly used, the term "complication" has a connotation of the unusual or unexpected. But many problems that arise postoperatively are not unexpected and are more accurately described as "side effects". Similar to esophagitis associated with mediastinal irradiation or alopecia secondary to treatment with antineoplastic drugs.

Complications in the true sense are local problems which, avoidably or otherwise, are causally related to the technical conduct of the surgical procedure.

These distinctions should be borne in mind during our discussion of postoperative problems. A total of 83 "complications" of various kinds occurred in 67 of the 206 patients who underwent 212 operations.

Cardiac Problems

Transient atrial fibrillation is one of the most common cardiac rhythm disturbances that followed pulmonary resections in our series. In 12 patients the arrhythmia occurred as an isolated event; in 6 others it was associated with other abnormalities (Table 27).

The incidence of atrial fibrillation in the pneumonectomized patients (10 of 72 = 14%) was twice as high as in patients who had lobectomies (9 of 122 = 7%).

Looking back at the preoperative findings, we see that most of these patients displayed abnormal pulmonary hemodynamics during exercise, and that most had essentially normal ECGs.

With three exceptions, the patients were treated with digitalis for several days prior to surgery. We are unable to provide data on degrees of saturation, which may not always have been within the therapeutic range.

Atrial fibrillation occurring de novo after surgery was treated in most cases with increased doses of intravenous digitalis. The onset of atrial fibrillation on the first or second postoperative day enabled us to continue with infusion therapy and instrumental monitoring of ECG, central venous pressure, and arterial pressure. Four patients received quinidine, and one received Verapamil. Only one patient required electrocardioversion because of severe hypotension.

In one 55-year-old man (B. K.) a relatively tachycardiac atrial fibrillation (110/min) persisted after a left pneumonectomy despite the use of electroversion and all available pharmacologic measures. Even so, the patient was able to work for another 6½ years and died 7 years after surgery from hemoptysis secondary to a recurrent tumor (squamous cell carcinoma) in the right main bronchus.

The literature, too, points to atrial fibrillation or atrial flutter as the most common cardiac dysrhythmia following pulmonary surgery [29, 93, 138, 172, 297, 342]. A review of the literature by Kirsh [172] showed that while atrial fibrillation is a relatively rare complication in patients under 50 years of age, it affects up to 30% of patients over 60. In addition, patients with preexisting heart disease are at particularly high risk for development of atrial fibrillation in the

Table 27. Postoperative atrial fibrillation

Patient	Op.	RC	ECG	Preop. digit.	HR	Therapy	Course
a) Isolated							
1. B.K., 55	P	+	nor	+	130	Digit. ↑	Established
2. B.W., 58	P	+	nor	+	140	Digit. ↑	Spont. conv.
3. B.H., 62	P	+	nor	+	140	Digit. ↑	Spont. conv.
4. D.J., 65	P	nor	LVH	+	160	Electroversion	
5. G.A., 65	P	nor	nor	+	140	Digit. ↑	Spont. conv.
6. H.A., 58	L	++	nor	+	100	Quinidine	Spont. conv.
7. H.B., 69	L	0	nor	0	150	Digit. new	Spont. conv.
8. L.E., 53	P	++	LVH	+	120	Digit. ↑	Spont. conv.
9. R.R., 72	L	+	REPOL	+	170	Digit. ↑	Spont. conv.
10. S.K., 61	P	0	nor	+	140	Digit. ↑ quin.	Spont. conv.
11. S.H., 52	P	nor	nor	0	150	Digit. new	Spont. conv.
12. W.G., 65	L	+	nor	+	150	Digit. ↑ quin.	Spont. conv.
b) Combined with other disorders							
13. D.W., 66	P	+	REPOL	+	140	Verapamil	Spont. conv.
(Klebsiella pneumonia, 5 days' ventilation, 3 wks in hospital)							
14. F.K., 74	BL	+	nor	+	130	Ditit. ↑	Spont. conv.
(17 day's chest drainage for bronchiolar fistula)							
15. G.A., 68	L	+	nor	+	150	Digit. ↑	Spont. conv.
(purulent bronchitis)							
16. K.K., 56	P	++	REPOL	+	120	Digit. ↑	Spont. conv.
(transient left hemisyndrome on day 5, pneumonia)							
17. T.P., 63	L	+	nor	+	140	Digit. ↑	Spont. conv.
(sputum retention, 12 days' ventilation, tracheotomy)							
18. S.J., 61	L	0	nor	0	150	Digit. new	Spont. conv.
(gastric bleeding, gangrene of toes, bacteremia, death from hemorrhage)							
19. F.N., 74	BL	+	VES	+	140	Digit. ↑ quin.	Spont. conv.
(resp. failure with sputum retention, ventilation, tracheotomy)							

RC: Right heart catheterization
+: Abnormal function during exercise
++: Exertional failure/active hypertension
0: No examination
nor: Normal
LVH: Evidence of left ventricular hypertrophy
REPOL: Repolarization defect
Digit. ↑: Increase in digitalis dosage
P: Pneumonectomy
L: Lobectomy
BL: Bilobectomy

postoperative period. Ungeheuer and Hartel [342] stress the predominance of this complication after pneumonectomy as compared with lobectomy. Johansson et al. [157] report an incidence of 46% after pneumonectomy versus 13% after partial lung resections.

Various causes have been postulated to account for the occurrence of atrial fibrillation after resective pulmonary surgery. Kraft-Kinz et al. [175] suggest that mediastinal displacement has causal significance. These authors noted a decline in the incidence of atrial fibrillation when the negative pressure in the pneumonectomy cavity was equalized.

Several authors have emphasized the value of digitalis in promoting spontaneous conversion to sinus rhythm [93, 138, 172, 342], though in some cases the drug must be combined with quinidine before this effect is obtained [297].

Digitalis also plays a leading role in efforts to *prevent* atrial fibrillation. Prophylactic digitalis remains a controversial therapy, however. A range of attitudes exist between outright rejection [297], selective utilization according to age or cardiac function [138, 342], and routine use [175]. Comparative studies by Shields and Ujiki [303] and Wheat and Burford [357] point to the benefits of preoperative digitalis in a wide range of patients. Kirsh et al. [172] recommend it for all patients who have preexisting cardiac disease.

In view of the age correlation that is apparent in the literature and in our own observations (Table 27), we tend to favor the liberal use of digitalis therapy. In patients over 50 years of age, we routinely initiate preoperative digitalis regardless of the results of hemodynamic tests. Younger patients are given digitalis only if function tests are abnormal.

Only two more patients were noted to have other significant cardiac problems. One patient, a 68-year-old man (S. A.), developed refractory ventricular premature beats with short bouts of ventricular tachycardia and second and third degree AV block following a lobectomy. He was hospitalized a total of three weeks. Enzyme studies raised the suspicion of myocardial infarction, but this could not be confirmed by ECG because of preexisting left bundle branch block. The patient died in 1984 without autopsy, more than 10 years after the pulmonary resection.

A fatal outcome occurred in a 48-year-old man (K. H.) with squamous cell carcinoma (postoperative stage III: T2, N2, M0) who developed bradycardia with a third degree AV block and arterial hypotension 4 hours after a radical resection of the left upper lobe. The patient required external cardiac massage, and isoproterenol was administered. These measures established an acceptable nodal rhythm with satisfactory hemodynamics. Ventricular fibrillation ensued one hour later, and efforts at resuscitation were futile. Before operation, this patient was noted to have right ventricular dysfunction with signs of lateral ischemia in the ECG. Chest radiographs showed marked kyphosis and a prominent, elongated aorta. These findings contraindicated a pneumonectomy, which would have been preferred in a stage III case of this type. Autopsy disclosed moderate aortic stenosis with partial calcification of the aortic valve, eccentric left ventricular hypertrophy, and coronary artery sclerosis with no critical stenoses. In retrospect, insufficient attention was given to the cardiac pathology in this patient. An aortic murmur was not documented and possibly was obscured by overlying emphysema associated with kyphoscoliosis. Surgical therapy would not be advised in an acute situation of this type.

Respiratory Problems

Pulmonary difficulties after resective lung surgery are an even greater concern than cardiac problems. Despite the careful preparation of high-risk patients, the inability to cough effectively in the early postoperative period can lead to problems that affected approximately 10% of the patients operated in this series.

The clinical picture of postoperative respiratory distress is usually impressive, and the condition is easily diagnosed. At the onset coarse rales are heard over the trachea, and the patient makes ineffectual attempts to raise airway secretions. There is a marked progression of respiratory failure within the space of a few hours, typically accompanied by alternating periods of restlessness and apathy. The blockage of secretions in the major airways soon leads to the development of atelectases and then to acute bronchopneumonia.

With prompt recognition and treatment, the progression of respiratory failure can be halted with a minimum of intervention, provided the patient is reasonably cooperative. Usually, intensive physiotherapy is no longer adequate when frank respiratory distress exists. However, the repeated nasotracheal suctioning of airway secretions is an effective way of clearing central tracheobronchial passages. In favorable cases this will elicit a very strong cough reflex that will raise secretions from the lobar bronchi, which are not accessible to a blindly inserted catheter.

The selective aspiration of secretions with a fiberoptic bronchoscope is even more effective and is less traumatizing. While the use of a topical anesthetic will obtund the cough reflex, it also enables a systematic aspiration and the local application of secretolytic agents. The risk of critical hypoxia is less than with blind suctioning, and the procedure is less stressful.

If respiratory decompensation cannot be checked by this method, intubation and mechanical ventilation are unavoidable, and a poorer prognosis is implied.

Sputum Retention and Atelectasis

In nine patients sputum retention was uncomplicated by clinical or radiologic signs of bronchopneumonia and could be managed by the relatively noninvasive measure of suctioning. Endoscopic aspiration was the method of choice (Table 28). Some of the patients responded satisfactorily to intensive physiotherapy and postural drainage.

All patients with retained secretions had undergone lobectomies. Most were upper lobectomies, and two were sleeve resections. In the sleeve operations, sputum retention was the result of a mechanical stenosis caused by mucosal edema at the anastomosis and by a lingering disturbance of mucociliary function. Most patients had a severe or very severe obstructive defect of lung function that had been intensively treated prior to surgery.

In one patient (case 9 in the table) endotracheal suctioning was effective for only a few days. We found that this was due to a tendency of the right main stem bronchus to become kinked. This 58-year-old man had a predominantly restrictive defect of ventilatory function associated with preexisting silicotuberculosis. Seven weeks earlier he had undergone surgery elsewhere for a squamous cell carcinoma. Histologic findings showed that the segmentectomy was inadequate to provide complete elimination of the upper lobar tumor. The apical segment of the lower lobe also had to be sacrificed at reoperation. Subsequent recurrent atelectasis of the residual lung, which was due partly to mechanical causes, necessitated a residual pneumonectomy three weeks later.

Table 28. Sputum retention and atelectasis

No.	Pat.	Age	Resection	Preoperative lung function	Preop. antibiot. therapy	Course
1.	B.K.	59	Rt. UL sleeve	Obstruction + +	Yes	ETA successful
2.	E.O.	63	Left UL	Obstruction + + (β blocker)	Yes	ETA successful
3.	G.A.	68	Left LL	Normal	No	ETA successful
4.	G.A.	58	Left UL	Obstruction +	Yes	ETA successful (prolonged air fistula)
5.	H.S.	66	Left UL	Obstruction + +	No (steroids)	ETA successful
6.	H.H.	73	Left UL sleeve	Obstruction + +	Yes	ETA successful
7.	L.F.	74	Rt. UL	Obstruction + +	Yes	ETA successful
8.	M.H.	60	Rt. UL	Obstruction (+)	No	ETA successful
9.	W.K.	58	Rt. UL & seg. 6	Restriction +	No	Recurrent atelectasis/residual pneumonectomy

UL = Upper lobe
LL = Lower lobe
ETA = Endotracheal aspiration

(+) = Mild
\+ = Moderate
\+ + = Severe

Postoperative Bronchopneumonia

Seven patients developed bronchopneumonia after surgery (Table 29). The criteria for this diagnosis were positive radiography, fever, leukocytosis, and significant bacteriologic findings in tracheal secretions. An early onset was common to all cases. Only one patient responded satisfactorily to repeated bronchoscopic tracheobronchial toilet combined with specific antibiotic therapy. All other patients required reintubation and several days of ventilatory support because of global respiratory failure. One patient died on the 10th postoperative day after a bronchopleural fistula developed while he was on the ventilator.

Klebsiella and Pseudomonas were the pathogenic organisms most frequently isolated from affected patients.

If we compare this group of patients with the patients who had "uncomplicated" retention of secretions, we find that pneumonectomies and bilobectomies were predominant in the bronchopneumonia group, but that, surprisingly, these patients were less apt to show serious function impairment during preoperative testing.

In explaining the occurrence of life-threatening pulmonary complications in patients who had a better initial functional status on average, we must assume that other factors were present which lowered resistance to pulmonary infection. Thus, four patients had an advanced tumor stage, and in two cases this

Table 29. Postoperative bronchopneumonia

No.	Pat.	Age	Operation	Preop. lung function	Therapy/course	Bacteriology
1.	B.R.	66	Pneumon.	Normal	Reintubated day 2 Stump leak day 4 Death day 10	Klebsiella, E. coli, Pseudomonas
2.	D.W.[a]	66	Pneumon.	Normal	Reintubated day 3 Discharged 3 wks. postop.	Klebsiella
3.	F.K.	74	Bilobect.	Obstruc.	Extended primary ventilation, tracheotomy Discharged after 3 months	Pseudomonas
4.	R.M.	56	Bilobect.	Restric.	Reintubated day 4 Discharged 3 wks. postop.	Pseudomonas
5.	S.M.	65	Pneumon.	Normal	Bronchoscop. aspiration	Klebsiella
6.	S.C.	65	Lobect.	Obstruc.	Reintubated 2× days 2 and 6 Discharged 3 wks. postop.	Pseudomonas
7.	T.P.	63	Lobect. (sleeve)	Normal	Reintubated day 3 Tracheotomy Discharged 4 wks. postop.	Klebsiella

[a] No preoperative antibiotics

was combined with paraneoplastic syndrome (osteoarthropathy). Two patients suffered from insulin-dependent diabetes, complicated in one case by renal failure secondary to phenacetin abuse.

Patient 3 in Table 29 had a particularly unfavorable initial status, as described below:

Patient F. K., 74 years of age: Squamous cell carcinoma of the right upper lobe with abscess formation, fetid sputum. Cardiac arrest occurred at initial thoracotomy (suspected dextran allergy). Open resuscitation was successful, and the procedure was terminated without resection. Recovery was uneventful, and a palliative bilobectomy was performed on the following day. Spontaneous respiration was inadequate, and so ventilatory support was continued postoperatively. Pneumonia and recurrent atrial fibrillation ensued. Repeated attempts were made to wean the patient from the ventilator, with hypoxic circulatory arrest occurring 4 weeks postoperatively accompanied by transient hemisyndrome. Patient was discharged at 3 months and survived an additional 16 months at home. Autopsy was not performed.

Cases of severe bronchopneumonia, which are not listed in Table 29, developed as *secondary* complications in 5 patients. Two cases had a fatal outcome. These involved pulmonary infections that were not the indication for ventilation, but arose only after the patient had been placed on the ventilator; these cases are discussed elsewhere in greater detail.

Postoperative Hemoptysis

A peculiar postoperative complication occurred in a 51-year-old man (S. L.) in whom an adenocarcinoma of the left upper lobe had been extirpated by lobectomy. The patient had a history of tuberculosis with persistent residua in the apices of both lungs. For this reason we initiated tuberculostatic therapy with ethambutol/isoniazid before surgery and maintained the drug postoperatively. On day 8 the patient collapsed with acute hemoptysis, aspiration of blood, and subsequent hypoxemic circulatory arrest. The patient was successfully resuscitated by intubation, ventilation, and closed-chest cardiac massage. Immediate fiberoptic bronchoscopy identified the contralateral upper lobe as the source of the hemorrhage. During transport to emergency surgery, there was a recurrence of profuse bleeding that necessitated an emergency thoracotomy without aseptic precautions. The second lobectomy was well tolerated, and the postoperative course was uneventful. Pathologic examination showed the bleeding source to be a posttuberculous upper lobar bronchiectasis. Two years later the patient died from a functionally inoperable squamous cell carcinoma (after primary adenocarcinoma!), the immediate cause of death being a fatal hemorrhage through a communication between the esophagus and pulmonary artery.

The Role of Antibiotic Therapy

Our approach to the use of antibiotics should be discussed briefly in connection with respiratory difficulties. Aside from a few carcinomas associated with abscess formation or poststenotic pneumonia, our patients did not suffer from *acute* airway infections. Nevertheless, the majority were treated with antibiotics prior to surgery. This is because pulmonary resections involve the opening of large bronchi and therefore are not aseptic operations in the strict sense [188]. In addition, patients with lung carcinoma tend to be elderly, most have coexisting tumor-independent pulmonary disease, and many are debilitated and immune-compromised by their cancer [299].

Bronchoscopy demonstrated the presence of chronic bronchitis in more than 90% of our surgical patients. There is no question that abstinence from smoking, secretolytic drugs, inhalation therapy, and physiotherapy are beneficial in such cases, provided the raising of airway secretions is not blocked by tumor stenosis. In practice, however, these measures are time-consuming and often are difficult to implement properly on an outpatient basis. This is why antibiotics have become a more or less routine preliminary to lung cancer surgery.

Systematic sputum examinations have shown that Hemophilus influenzae, pneumococci, staphylococci, and Enterobacter species are the organisms most commonly found in the bronchial secretions of bronchitis patients. Liebig et al. [193] have shown that tetracycline strongly reduces all of these organisms during the first two days of therapy, but that counts of Enterobacter species, especially *E. coli*, increase again if the drug is maintained for a longer period.

When bronchial smears and mucosal biopsies were taken intraoperatively for bacteriologic study, bacteria (staphylococci and a few Klebsiella) were cultured four times more frequently in patients who did not receive preoperative antibiotics. Pleural empyemas were significantly less common after tetracycline therapy, but only if the drug had been initiated two days before surgery.

Other authors recommend penicillin [22] or penicillin/streptomycin [138] for the prophylaxis of postoperative infectious complications. Because tetracyclines are active against gram-positive and gram-negative organisms and thus against staphylococci and pneumococci, Vibramycin was the drug of choice in our population. Of course if an infectious complication arises, it is necessary to modify the antibiotic to allow for drug resistance. We alternately used trimethoprim/sulfamethoxazol (Bactrim), ampicillin, or amoxycillin depending on bacteriologic results in samples obtained at bronchoscopy.

As we have shown, the rate of postoperative infections in our series was low, with only a 3.4% incidence of bronchopneumonia. On the other hand, it is typical of the preoperative antibiotic therapy used that the predominant causal agents of these complicating infections were Klebsiella, *E. coli,* and Pseudomonas, which can fill the "ecologic nitch" left by Hemophilus influenzae. This is why antibiotics active against the problem organisms were not used preoperatively in patients who had chronic bronchitis.

Cerebral Complications

While neurologic complications relating to pulmonary surgery are rarely mentioned in the literature [66], they played a role in the postoperative course of our patients that was comparable to that of bronchopneumonia. It seems appropriate, therefore, to present brief case reports on the seven patients in our series (all males) who manifested cerebral complications after surgery.

1. C. A., 56 years of age: *Lobectomy.* Arm paresis on 2nd postoperative day with no impairment of consciousness. CT scan of head normal. No residua at discharge 2 weeks postoperatively. Patient survived 6 years and 3 months without further cerebral incidents. Cause of death was progressive adenocarcinoma. Autopsy showed no cerebral pathology.
2. K. K., 56 years of age: *Left pneumonectomy.* Atrial fibrillation on 2nd postoperative day, spontaneous conversion. Left hemisyndrome 3 days later. Normal carotid angiogram. Symptoms regressed until discharge at 2 weeks. Patient survived 3½ years. Clinical cause of death was myocardial infarction; autopsy was not performed.
3. M. M., 60 years of age: *Right pneumonectomy.* Cerebrovascular accident on 2nd postoperative day with brief loss of consciousness and transient weakness on left side of body. Brain scan normal. Patient was discharged at 2 weeks, and died 5 months later from cardiac arrest. *Autopsy* showed metastatic tumor of ventricular septum with no cerebral pathology.
4. P. O., 57 years of age: *Right pneumonectomy.* Cerebrovascular accident with unconsciousness and apnea on 5th postoperative day. Left hemiplegia. Rapid recovery and complete regression of paralysis within 3 days. CT head scan normal. Discharged at 2 weeks postop. Mitral valve was replaced 5 years later without complications. Patient has survived 10 years.
5. G. K., 66 years of age: *Sleeve lobectomy* of right upper lobe. Cerebrovascular accident on 1st postoperative day with persistent unconsciousness. Intubation, ventilation, later tracheotomy. Secondary bronchopneumonia. EEG and brain scan consistent with metastasis in posterior cranial fossa. Death at 5 weeks from candidal sepsis. *Autopsy* showed extensive malacia of right hemisphere, probably from embolic occlusion of right middle cerebral artery.
6. J. T., 60 years of age: *Exploratory thoracotomy* for inoperable squamous cell carcinoma. Cerebrovascular accident 5 days postoperatively; unconsciousness, intubation and ventilation. Brain scan suspicious for mass lesion of left temporoparietal area. Death from car-

diac failure associated with coronary heart disease (history of MI 8 weeks preoperatively). *Autopsy* showed large metastasis in left occipital area.

7. K. R., 56 years of age: *Pneumonectomy*. Hematemesis on 1st postoperative day. Generalized seizure hours later. Intubation and ventilation. Brain scan suspicious for metastatic space-occupying lesion. Persistent spasmophilia. Bronchopneumonia developed on 4th postoperative day. Death on day 6 from respiratory failure and gastric bleeding. *Autopsy* showed malacia of putamen (at least 3 weeks old) and cerebral atrophy. Patient had history of unexplained episodes of dizziness.

With three fatal outcomes, cerebral complications contributed significantly to the overall mortality in this series. Except for the last patient, there was no anamnestic or – in surviving patients – catamnestic evidence to suggest that a prohibitive risk was present.

In five patients we must attribute cerebral symptoms to an embolic process which in four cases was benign and in one case led to extensive malacia. In one patient the cerebral complication possibly was related to intercurrent atrial fibrillation. Other possible causes are paradoxic emboli associated with a patent foramen ovale, and the dislodgement of left atrial parietal thrombi at the site of the pulmonary venous ligature. An exhaustive study of the patients' records was unable to confirm these hypotheses. We found no evidence of elevated central venous pressures or peripheral phlebitis. Hypoxic states also were excluded. Anticoagulation either had not been initiated in early postoperative cases or was not yet within the therapeutic range. Perfect anticoagulation was achieved in one patient (No. 4 above) who suffered a cerebrovascular accident on the fifth day after pneumonectomy.

In two patients who died, autopsy disclosed a preexisting pathologic condition which decompensated at approximately the time of the operation. One involved a previously asymptomatic brain metastasis, and the other involved an ischemic process with episodes of dizziness; neither condition had been given sufficient attention during preoperative evaluation.

Based on these experiences, we must ascribe ominous prognostic significance to any cerebral disturbances that arise in the postoperative period.

Intestinal Complications

Like cerebral disturbances, gastrointestinal problems are rarely mentioned as a complication of lung cancer surgery. Their incidence in the present series is low, yet their effect on the postoperative course can be profound, as illustrated by three observations:

1. K. R., 56 years of age (case 7 above): *Pneumonectomy*. Hematemesis on 1st postoperative day. It is possible that the massive gastric bleeding, through hemodynamic effects and acute transfusions, precipitated the generalized epileptic seizure that followed (operative death).
2. E. B., 69 years of age: *Lobectomy* for stage I oat cell carcinoma. On day 3 erosive gastritis with gastric bleeding not responsive to conservative measures. Truncal vagotomy and pyloroplasty were performed on same day, followed 10 days later by acute recurrence of bleeding (14th postop. day). Suture-ligation of ulcer and ligature of left gastric artery. Pneumonia (Proteus and Klebsiella) supervened. 16 days later the patient, who felt well and was ambulating, died from central pulmonary embolism (no anticoagulation). Autopsy showed no metastases from lung carcinoma.

3. H. A., 65 years of age: *Lobectomy.* Laparotomy on 5th postoperative day for acute abdomen: perforation of cecum. Oversewing was followed by subileus and ileus. Repeat laparotomy on day 10 with freeing of adhesions and cecostomy. Patient was discharged and readmitted 3 days later with acute abdomen. *Third* laparotomy 30 days after lung resection: cholecystectomy of gangrenous gallbladder. Further course complicated by bronchopneumonia. Death from terminal renal failure occurred 3½ months after cancer resection. Autopsy showed no metastases.
4. S. J., 61 years of age: *Middle lobectomy* for bronchioloalveolar carcinoma. Arterial occlusive disease; prior above-knee amputation of leg, gangrene of toes on opposite side. Diabetes. Chronic therapy with Voltaren and Zyloric. Gastric bleeding on 3rd postoperative day, tachycardiac atrial fibrillation converted with digitalis, fever: streptococcal bacteremia with now moist gangrene of toes 3–5. Patient died in acute circulatory failure on 6th postoperative day. Autopsy showed massive hemorrhage from multiple antral erosions.

As these cases illustrate, abdominal complications coinciding with major intrathoracic operations initiate a process, usually through secondary pulmonic infection, that can culminate in total failure.

Thromboembolic Complications: Pulmonary Embolism

Acute central pulmonary embolism is a dreaded complication of any surgical procedure. In no other type of operation it is so consistently lethal, however, as after pulmonary resections and especially after pneumonectomies.

As a complication of nonthoracic surgery, acute pulmonary embolism leading to circulatory collapse has a high mortality rate, and a successful embolectomy is possible only in favorable circumstances. After pneumonectomy, the chance of saving a patient with pulmonary embolism is very small. We know of no case where an embolism of this type was successfully treated by embolectomy.

In an effort to prevent this complication, we routinely employ thromboembolism prophylaxis at our center. During the period of our study, the regimen consisted in the administration of 500 ml of 6% dextran during the operation and again on the 1st postoperative day. The first dose of dicoumarin (Marcoumar) was given orally on the 2nd postoperative day with the intent of achieving a prothrombin value of 25% as rapidly as possible. In the absence of special indications for its continuance, anticoagulant therapy was discontinued when the patient was fully ambulatory and ready to be discharged. Today we do not hesitate to perform mediastinoscopies as well as lung resections under continued, preoperative coumarin therapy in the therapeutically active range.

Personal Observations

Five fatal pulmonary embolisms occurred in this series: two each following lobectomy and left pneumonectomy, and one following right pneumonectomy. In two cases the diagnosis was based on clinical evaluation and in three cases on postmortem findings.

One case already has been discussed in connection with gastrointestinal complications. The patient died from a fulminant pulmonary embolism 30 days after undergoing a lobectomy and two laparotomies. Hemorrhagic complications in this patient contraindicated anticoagulation, and so the connection with pulmonary surgery was indirect.

The pulmonary embolisms presented differently in the four remaining patients:

1. W. K., 61 years of age: Lobectomy of the left lower lobe for squamous cell carcinoma. Prolonged intubation and ventilation for obstructive lung disease without a strict indication. Infusion therapy was still being maintained on the 4th postoperative day. Central venous pressure 3 h before death was 4 cm H_2O. Cause of death was acute circulatory failure secondary to central pulmonary embolism. Autopsy showed calf-vein thrombosis. Thromboembolism prophylaxis: Dextran at operation and on 1st postoperative day; coumarin was not administered.
2. K. W., 65 years of age: Radical left pneumonectomy for squamous cell carcinoma. Nephrotic syndrome interpreted as paraneoplastic. Persistent leg edema and hypalbuminemia after surgery. Transferred at 15 days for further renal evaluation. Death occurred 37 days after pneumonectomy. Thromboembolism prophylaxis: Dextran at operation and on 1st postoperative day; Marcoumar started on 2nd postoperative day. Anticoagulation was discontinued 4 days after transferral (14 days before death). Autopsy showed femoral vein thrombosis.
3. B. A., 64 years of age: Left pneumonectomy for adenocarcinoma. Death from pulmonary embolism (clinical) on 2nd postoperative day. Prophylaxis: dextran and 1st dose of Marcoumar with prothrombin of 64%. Autopsy was refused.
4. R. D., 59 years of age: Radical right pneumonectomy. Acute circulatory death on 2nd postoperative day. Prophylaxis was not administered. Autopsy was refused.

Taking a critical look at the brief case reports presented above, we can find plausible reasons for some of the postoperative pulmonary embolisms that occurred. It is difficult to say whether the earlier initiation of anticoagulant therapy in cases 1 and 3 could have prevented pulmonary embolism. In case 1 it seems apparent that "overtreatment" and delayed ambulation contributed to the thromboembolic complication.

It is noteworthy that from 1975 to 1978 and in subsequent years, no additional case of fatal pulmonary embolism has occurred in our surgical patients. The reason for this is not entirely clear, but presumably it relates to the shortening of postoperative intensive care: Patients are extubated within hours after surgery, infusions are seldom maintained longer than 24 h, and patients are ambulated on the first postoperative day.

Reports vary greatly on the incidence of massive and fatal pulmonary embolisms following lung resections. A survey conducted by Clarke [54] indicated a frequency between 0% and 4%. In a total of 11300 resections, Clarke received reports of 134 fatal pulmonary embolisms, corresponding to 1.2%. These embolisms accounted for 14% of the overall mortality. R. A. Smith [313] reports 38 autopsy-verified pulmonary embolisms in 1200 resections, corresponding to an incidence of over 3% and accounting for 43% of postoperative deaths. The same author notes that autopsy disclosed central pulmonary embolism in over 90% of cases given a clinical diagnosis of acute circulatory death. Fryjordet and Klevmark [88] state that pulmonary embolism accounts for 27% of primary mortality. Embolism-linked mortality in the German literature, according to Ungeheuer and Hartel [342], ranges between 12% and 28.5%. An analysis of postoperative complications by Huth and Diwok [145] in 221 lung resections (122 for carcinoma) does not contain a single case of pulmonary embolism.

Although it has been demonstrated that thrombus formation in the stump of the pulmonary artery can precipitate a fatal pulmonary embolism [322], this would occur mainly in right-sided pneumonectomies and never in lobectomies, and presumably is extremely rare as a causative mechanism [172]. According to Clarke [54], it is significant that fatal pulmonary embolisms are ten times more frequent after lung cancer resections than after resections for benign disease. It remains unclear whether this relates to the malignant disease itself or to the average higher patient age and coexisting cardiac burden.

Surgical Complications

In this section we shall examine complications that relate to the technical aspects of pulmonary resections. It should be kept in mind that preexistent organ changes frequently play a role in the etiology of these complications.

Bronchopleural Fistula

Bronchopleural fistula, known also as bronchial leak, stump leak or stump insufficiency, is the best known and also one of the most dangerous local complications of resective lung surgery [22].

In 194 pulmonary resections, 5 bronchopleural fistulas occurred. Four occurred in a total of 72 pneumonectomies (5.5%), and 1 in a total of 122 partial lung resections (0.8%). This complication contributed very little to operative mortality, however.

Bronchopleural Fistula After Pneumonectomy

1. D. M., 60 years of age: Extended left pneumonectomy. Preoperative antibiotics given for poststenotic pneumonia. "Acute pulmonary edema" (Fig. 16 b) developed on day of scheduled discharge (13 days postop.): bronchopleural fistula, reoperation, closure. Mechanical ventilation for respiratory insufficiency. After 8 days on ventilator, signs of fistula reappeared. To avoid the infected left pleural cavity, a sternotomy was performed and the fistula was closed through a transpericardial approach [30]. Patient was discharged with continuous drainage of persistent empyema for 7 months. Fatal myocardial infarction occurred 20 months after the primary operation. Autopsy showed a large recurrent tumor with involvement of the left coronary branches.
2. E. H., 58 years of age: Radical right pneumonectomy done as an emergency operation for hemoptysis. Antibiotics were not administered preoperatively. Bifocal large cell carcinoma was removed. Bronchial leak developed on 10th postoperative day: aspiration, dyspnea. At reoperation stump was freshened and resutured. Suction irrigation with chloramine solution was maintained for 20 days. Stump healed without empyema. Patient later underwent surgery and radiotherapy for brain metastases and has survived for more than 5 years.
3. K. G., 66 years of age: Extended right pneumonectomy, infiltration of vena cava by poorly differentiated squamous cell carcinoma. Fever and leukocytosis at 12 days postoperatively, purulent material aspirated from pneumonectomy cavity. Reoperation and drainage on day 14. A 1-mm fistula was oversewn and covered (primary suture at level of trachea). Suction irrigation with chloramine solution. Patient was discharged without empyema 6 weeks postoperatively. Death occurred 3 months later from tumor cachexia, pulmonary emboli in the left lower lobe, and postinfarction pneumonia. Autopsy showed intact tracheal suture and no empyema.
4. B. R., 66 years of age: Radical right pneumonectomy for squamous cell carcinoma with ipsilateral mediastinal metastases. Sputum retention and global insufficiency after surgery.

Ventilatory support started on 2nd postoperative day for bronchopneumonia with mixed flora (see Table 29). Soft-tissue emphysema developed on day 4 during positive-pressure ventilation with inspiratory pressures up to 40 cm H_2O. Bronchoscopy showed needle tract fistula at bronchial suture line. Patient was considered too ill for reintervention. Death from bronchopneumonia (clinical and autopsy) occurred on 10th postoperative day. Autopsy showed small (< 1-mm) stump fistula, also a second squamous cell carcinoma and small peripheral adenocarcinoma of the left upper lobe (triple carcinoma).

Bronchopleural Fistula After Lobectomy

5. P. E., 37 years of age: Lower bilobectomy (right) for squamous cell carcinoma. Hemoptysis, persistent air leak through chest tube, and subfebrile temperatures on 11th postoperative day. Rethoracotomy and secondary suture. Patient developed bronchopneumonia, required prolonged ventilatory support, was discharged 7 weeks after primary resection. Fatal hemorrhage occurred 14 months later. Autopsy showed erosion of right pulmonary artery by recurrent tumor.

All cases but the last were characterized by an advanced stage of local tumor growth. The need for a complete resection may conflict with the requirement of preserving the blood supply in the area of the suture line. Our technique for closure of the bronchial stump employs an uninterrupted mattress suture followed by a continuous over-and-over suture. Interrupted sutures may also be used when the main bronchus has been transected at the level of the trachea. The suture material in this series consisted of 0 chromic catgut for main bronchi and 00 chromic catgut for lobar bronchi. Anastomoses after sleeve resections were sutured with 3-0 or 4-0 Prolene. Today we prefer to use synthetic, absorbable material for stump closures and for anastomoses. Even coverage of the stump with wide-based pericardial or pleural flaps has not entirely eliminated the risk of suture line leak.

Kirsh et al. [172] state that the incidence of bronchial leak was as high as 28% in the first two decades of resective surgery. Since then the rate has fallen to approximately 3% [27, 342]. Besides improvements in technique, this decline is due largely to the development of compatible suture materials and the use of double-lumen tubes for differential ventilation during surgery. With rare exceptions, we have used Robert Shaw tubes for the intraoperative ventilation of our patients since 1973.

The most dangerous bronchial leak is that which follows a pneumonectomy. Ungeheuer and Hartel [342] state that the mortality from that complication was as high as 48% in 1968. Harmon et al. [113] report that a series of 351 pneumonectomies in 1976 included 29 cases of bronchopleural fistula (8%) with 5 associated deaths (17%).

The causes of bronchial leak may relate to technical deficiencies – a traumatizing suture, a long bronchial stump that pools infectious secretions, denudation of the stump and distal trachea, and inadequate coverage. It is uncertain what advantage is gained from the use of an automatic stapling device. As with conventional sutures, technical experience is required.

In a clinical comparison, Peterfy and Calabrese [266] found that staples were associated with fewer bronchopleural fistulas than manually placed chromic catgut sutures (1% vs. 3%), but they also point out that stapling is not recommended when the bronchial lumen has to be inspected.

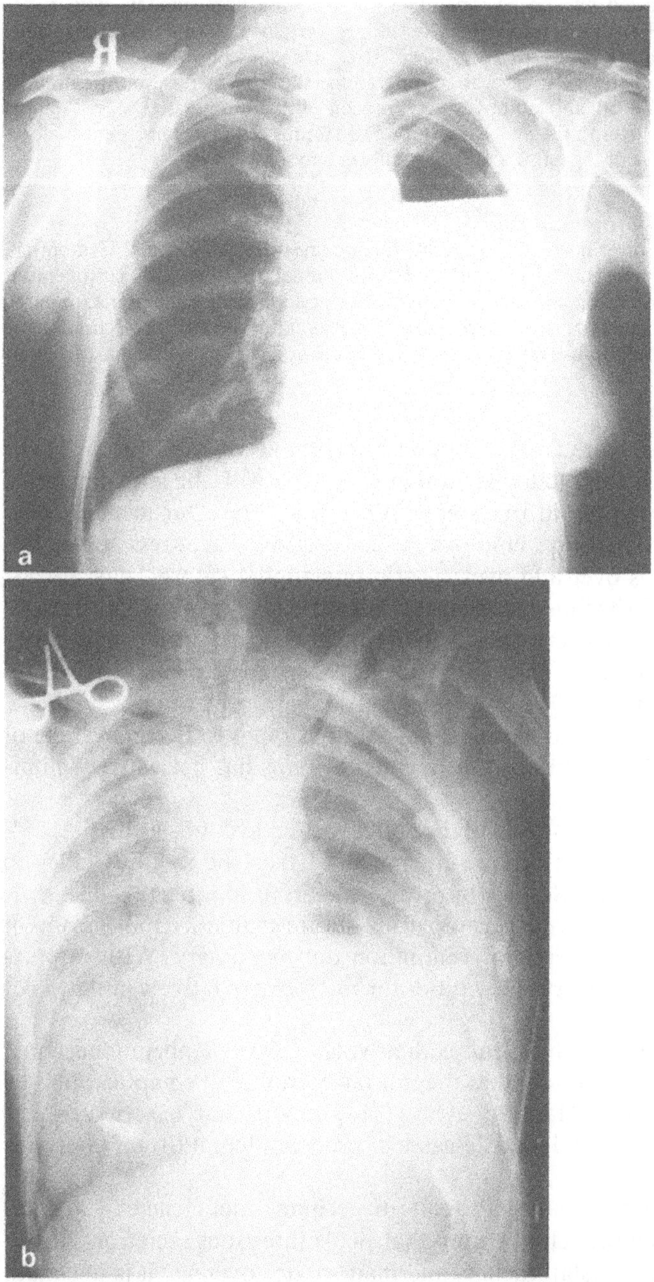

Fig. 16. a Radiographic sequence showing development of stump leak after left pneumonectomy (patient D. M., m., 60 years of age, pT3, N1, M0 adenocarcinoma with atrial invasion). PA chest radiograph taken 12 days after extended pneumonectomy shows typical presentation of seropneumothorax. The patient felt well. **b** Same patient. Chest radiograph made in supine state 7 h later with clinical picture of hemorrhaging lung edema, hypoxemia, and shock. Compared with **a,** light area to the left and diffuse density on the right: massive aspiration of serothorax

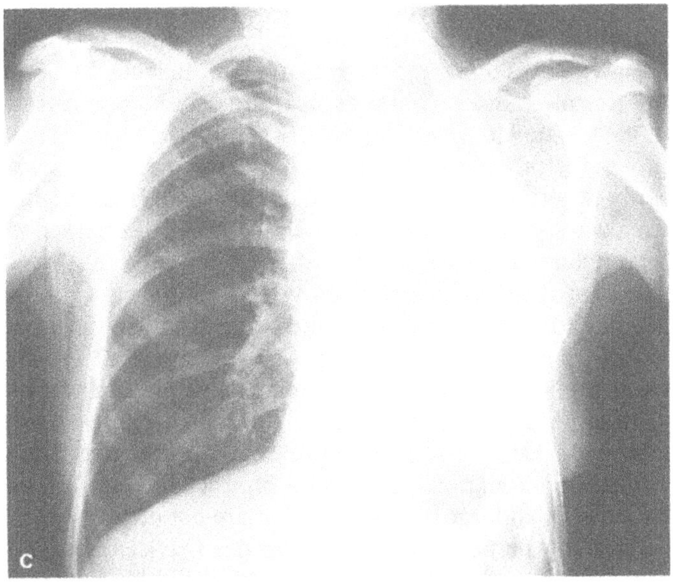

Fig. 16. c Condition after transsternal closure of bronchopleural fistula (second reoperation)

Studies by Smith et al. [312] showed that the mode of bronchial healing is not affected by the closure technique. Definitive healing occurred in two-thirds of cases with or without partial dehiscence of the suture line. One-third of cases went on to complete dehiscence, with the margins covered by surrounding tissue and epithelialized by bronchial mucosa.

Extensive skeletization proximal to the stump suture with sacrifice of vascular tissue is occasionally necessitated by a tumor that has infiltrated the peribronchial and peritracheal tissues [172]. Residual tumor at the line of resection has also been implicated as a cause of bronchopleural fistula.

Intrinsic causes include tissue damage resulting from previous irradiation, and fragility of the airway cartilages with tearing of the pars membranacea. The latter is especially common in the elderly.

A bronchopleural fistula can develop at any time during the first two weeks after surgery. Small fistulas are characterized by a light blood-staining of the sputum. Fistulas of this type are not acutely life-threatening as a rule, but they may lead to empyema of the pneumonectomy cavity, in which a large volume of serous exudate provides an excellent culture medium for bacteria. With larger suture dehiscence, copious amounts of this fluid enter the airways and are aspirated into the intact contralateral lung, precipitating acute respiratory failure. The clinical picture is similar to that of acute pulmonary edema, as moist rales are audible over residual lung and a large amount of frothy sputum is produced (Fig. 16).

The primary step in the management of this complication is to position the patient on the operated side and, if necessary, remove residual effusions from the pneumonectomy cavity by aspiration. Borrie [32] recommends that this be followed by open evacuation and the institution of continuous drainage, and that thoracoplasty be performed as a late measure. Similar recommendations are given by Young and Perryman [368]. Belcher and Sturridge [22] state that the treatment of choice is a repeat thoracotomy with freshening and reclosure of the stump. However, Ungeheuer and Hartel [342] do not believe that this improves the prognosis. Because conservative treatment by drainage alone necessarily results in the development of early empyema requiring chronic drainage, we always strived for a "total correction" of postresection bronchopleural fistulas in our patients.

Urgent reintervention has proved to be the best approach for patients who are able to tolerate anesthesia and surgery. In two cases urgency was compelled by the dramatic clinical course. At reoperation we usually found considerable tissue proliferation around the bronchial suture that was helpful in effecting the reclosure. At this time we also debrided the pneumonectomy cavity and established suction irrigation to prevent empyema and thus spare the patient the burden of chronic infection and a protracted course of treatment. We believe, moreover, that large dehiscences that are not operatively corrected compromise survival by perpetuating a massive dead-space ventilation and exposing the bronchial tree of the remaining lung to contamination from the infectious focus of the empyema cavity.

Bronchioloalveolar Fistula (Parenchymal Fistula)

Bronchiolalveolar fistula is manifested by a persistent air leak through the intrapleural drainage catheter following a *partial* pulmonary resection. A prolonged air leak of this type is considered a benign complication after a lobectomy or segmentectomy. It is the product of an extremely common lesion of the residual pulmonary parenchyma that occurs in all segmentectomies and in many lobectomies where the pulmonary fissures are incomplete. Complete aerostatis can rarely be accomplished by operative means. This is a major reason why the pleural cavity should be drained with large-bore tubes, which can vent leaked respiratory air to the outside together with local secretions. This will ensure expansion of the residual parenchyma. Most parenchymal fistulas close spontaneously within a few days as the residual lobe becomes apposed to the chest wall, and fibrinous adhesions develop which occlude the air leak. This may not occur, however, if a large discrepancy exists between the residual lung and the chest cavity, as is the case in the early period following a right bilobectomy. Other reasons are inadequate drainage or marked emphysematous parenchymal lesions. The result is a persistent air leak with or without radiographic evidence of a partial pneumothorax. Differentiation from bronchopleural fistula is possible without bronchoscopy when the sputum is clear, leukocytes are not elevated, and the patient is nonfebrile.

Most affected patients belonged to the group that had severe preexisting obstructive lung disease. The average length of postoperative treatment, 10 to 14 days, was at times considerably increased by protracted drainage and extended clinical observation (Table 30). In some cases (especially case 8) prolonged hos-

Table 30. Bronchioloalveolar fistulas

No.	Pat.	Age	Resection	Contributing factors	Length of postop. treatment
1.	E.J.	49	Rt. LL	Emphysema	16 days
2.	F.K.	74	LL/ML	Small residual lung	20 days
3.	G.A.	58	Left UL	Emphysema	15 days
4.	M.E.	72	Left UL +chest wall	Emphysema	22 days
5.	M.F.	65	UL/ML	Small residual lung	24 days
6.	S.L.	62	Rt. LL	Emphysema	16 days
7.	S.W.	53	Rt. UL	–	30 days
8.	S.E.	68	Left UL	Emphysema	54 days
9.	S.C.	65	Rt. UL	Mech. ventilation Emphysema	29 days

pitalization was related to factors other than air leak or residual pneumothorax. It should be added that early in the study there was a tendency to use secondary drainage as a means of promoting complete expansion. These measures, and the practice of awaiting the absorption of a residual pneumothorax, led to greatly extended hospitalization times in a few cases.

Brooks [42] and Kirsh et al. [172] recommend that partial pneumothorax or any unusual air leak noted in the immediate postoperative period be managed by creating a pneumoperitoneum in order to elevate the diaphragm. Brooks recommends thoracoplasty for cases of more than 14 days' duration.

In the opinion of Belcher and Sturridge [22], drainage tubes may be removed at 3–4 weeks without risk of infection despite the presence of an active air fistula. To shorten treatment, however, consideration must be given to rethoracotomy and surgical closure of the fistula.

It has been our experience [75] that bronchioloalveolar fistula is best managed conservatively. In many cases drainage tubes may be removed in only 10–14 days if trial clamping does not provoke an excessive rise of intrathoracic pressure or pulmonary collapse. Most residual pneumothoraces are absorbed in a period of a few weeks to three months, rarely longer. Based on favorable experience, we believe that spontaneous absorption may be awaited on an outpatient basis.

As early as 1966 Barker et al. [16] and Silver et al. [309] reported frequent spontaneous recoveries. Contrary to our experience, empyema developed in 6% and 12% of cases, respectively. However, it must be considered that their series included a number of partial resections for inflammatory processes (tuberculosis, bronchiectases, etc.).

Recurrent Laryngeal and Phrenic Nerve Paresis

Postoperative deficits involving the recurrent laryngeal nerve or phrenic nerve qualify as complications only if the integrity of these nerves was not deliberately compromised to obtain a complete tumor resection.

In this sense we observed two instances of recurrent laryngeal nerve paresis, one on the left side and one on the right, following ipsilateral pneumonectomies. The right-sided paresis reversed over a period of six months.

In no case has this complication led to secondary respiratory difficulties in the early postoperative period by impairing the ability to expel secretions by coughing.

One case of right-sided phrenic nerve paresis occurred in a patient who had been operated on for inflow statis with an unknown tumor histology. An inoperable small cell undifferentiated carcinoma was found, and surgery was limited to the creation of a venoatrial shunt, which caused no apparent trauma to the phrenic nerve. The paresis did not significantly affect respiratory function.

Rare Surgical Complications

Closed Chest-Wall Dehiscence After Pneumonectomy

Dehiscence of the chest wall occurred after a left pneumonectomy in a muscular, 39-year-old man whose general health was good. One week after surgery, a bulging of the posterolateral thoracic soft tissues was noted each time the patient coughed. The external wound was healing well, showed no signs of irritation, and there were no systemic signs of infection. Treatment consisted in placing a large pad over the thoracotomy site and securing it with a semielastic band. Borrie [32] attributes the phenomenon to a disruption of the intercostal layer. In our case hospitalization was prolonged by one week. Late follow-up showed no objective signs of detrimental effects from this complication.

Intraoperative Hemorrhage

Intraoperative hemorrhage becomes a complication only if it is uncontrollable or causes irreversible damage before it can be controlled. In two series of 96 and 91 pneumonectomies, Young and Perryman [368] report 1 death and 3 deaths, respectively, from intraoperative or perioperative hemorrhage.

One such event occurred in our series and resulted in death. The circumstances surrounding the hemorrhage, however, were unusual. The patient had undergone an incomplete carcinoma resection by left lower lobectomy at another clinic. The adequacy of the resection was not confirmed by frozen section examinations, and the bronchial margin was involved by tumor, necessitating postoperative radiation at a curative dose of 6000 rads. The patient was referred to us 14 months later for hemoptysis associated with a central tumor recurrence. At operation we found very extensive adhesions of the residual lung that were continuous with an area of tumor infiltration toward the posterior mediastinum. Even before resectability could be definitively assessed, the tumor-bearing wall of the descending aorta ruptured, causing a massive hemorrhage that led to circulatory arrest. The proximal aorta was snared and clamped, but the patient could not be saved. Based on this experience, we may conclude that thoracic reintervention after therapeutic irradiation is not advised, at least in cases where the postirradiation interval is comparable to that in our example. A previous thoracotomy alone or previous irradiation with a short interval alone is not considered a contraindication.

Postoperative Hemorrhage
Postoperative hemorrhage is not a complication specific to pulmonary surgery, but its occurrence after lung surgery has a special significance. This is because bleeding from the central vessels caused by the slipping of a ligature or loosening of a suture usually cannot be controlled in time if the chest has already been closed. The thoracic cavity exerts no pressure that could offer resistance to the hemorrhage. Knowledge of this danger should prompt particular care during closure of the large vascular stumps. Yet fatal postoperative hemorrhages are cited in the literature as a cause of operative mortality. Huth and Diwok [145], for example, report 2 deaths in 221 pulmonary resections. Wilkins and Saita (1983) counted 3 fatal hemorrhages in their review of 336 resections performed from 1961 to 1970, prompting them to recommend that the pulmonary artery stump be closed with a vascular suture rather than ligated, especially after pneumonectomy.

A more frequent cause of postoperative hemorrhage is lesions of small, usually arterial vessels of the chest wall or diaphragm, or bleeding from bronchial arteries that were inactive or unnoticed during the operation. Hemorrhages of this kind require that the chest be reopened. Brooks [42] states that rethoracotomy is indicated after a lobectomy when postoperative blood loss reaches 1000 ml.

We were forced to reopen the chest in a 71-year-old man who had undergone a left pneumonectomy. Instead of a severe isolated hemorrhage, we found only a diffuse extravasation from the dissection surfaces. The further course was uneventful, and postoperative care was not prolonged.

Cardiac Herniation
Cardiac herniation (or strangulation) denotes a condition in which the heart or a portion of it has prolapsed through a surgically created defect in the pericardium.

In our series this occurred in a 43-year-old woman who had undergone an extended left pneumonectomy for an invasive mucoepidermoid carcinoma. In this case almost the entire left side of the pericardium had to be included in the resection. Large defects of this kind are considered less problematic because true strangulation is not a danger. Nevertheless, the displacement of the heart that occurred when the patient was repositioned hampered right ventricular outflow, raised the right atrial pressure, and produced an intraatrial right-to-left shunt with marked arterial hypoxemia in the presence of a large, patent foramen ovale [118].

The complication was successfully managed by reopening the chest and covering the defect with parietal pleura.

Before 1975 there were only 40 reported cases of cardiac herniation, which had a 50% mortality (Refs. in Kirsh et al. [172]). Young and Perryman [368] report 2 additional cases that had fatal outcomes, and Arndt et al. [10] report an equal number that were successfully treated. The threat to life arises from an acute blockage of venous inflow, myocardial trauma, malignant dysrhythmias, or a combination of these problems. Pericardial defects necessarily occur when the great pulmonary vessels are divided within the pericardial sac, as in the resection of a central carcinoma, or when portions of the pericardium are resected because of tumor infiltration. Cardiac herniation is most effectively prevented by patching the defect with foreign (Teflon, dura mater) or autogenous material [32, 172, 368].

Postresection Empyema

Empyemas of the thoracic cavity after lung resections develop in an empty space or a space containing serous fluid. As we showed in our discussion of bronchioloalveolar fistula with incomplete expansion of the residual lung, empyema is rarely witnessed after *partial resections* for lung carcinoma. On the other hand, it is understandable that empyema might develop in the serofibrinous-filled cavity left by a *pneumonectomy.* This complication has been known since the first pneumonectomies were performed and once was a frequent complication of thoracic surgery in general [97, 98]. According to Kirsh et al. [172], the incidence of postpneumonectomy empyema has declined to about 5% for various reasons, one of the foremost being the use of antibiotic therapy.

Early Empyemas

Infections of the pneumonectomy cavity in the immediate postoperative period were mentioned earlier in connection with bronchial stump insufficiency. Only one patient developed a chronic empyema, which resolved after several months of continuous drainage (Fig. 16). In the remaining patients empyema could be prevented by closed suction irrigation of the bacteria-laden pleural cavity.

Late Empyemas

By definition, late empyema implies that the bronchial stump is intact, that there is no evidence of bronchial leak at any time in the postoperative period, and that at least two months have passed between operation and onset with no bridging symptoms such as leukocytosis or fever.

We saw empyemas of this type in two of our pneumonectomized patients:

1. B. K., 55 years of age (Fig. 17): Simple left pneumonectomy for a T3, N1, M0 squamous cell carcinoma. Postoperative course complicated by atrial fibrillation. Postoperative irradiation of the mediastinum. Three months later subfebrile temperatures; 1 week later high fever and empyema necessitans on the left side of the chest (*Staphylococcus aureus*). Empyema was evacuated by costotomy and closed suction irrigation; fluid sterile only after chloramine solution was used. Duration of treatment: 4 weeks. No reinfection occurred until death 7 years later from progression of tumor.
2. S. H., 52 years of age: Residual right pneumonectomy for recurrence of adenocarcinoma (T2, N1, M0) 11 years after primary resection. Postoperative course complicated by atrial fibrillation on day 4. Irradiation of the mediastinum discontinued because of jaundice (suspected hepatic metastases). Nine weeks postoperatively patient was ill with septic temperatures. Empyema was evacuated by basal thoracotomy and closed suction irrigation. After 2 weeks growth of *Staph. aureus* was still present; open drainage was instituted because the patient refused further hospitalization. Spontaneous obliteration and healing ensued

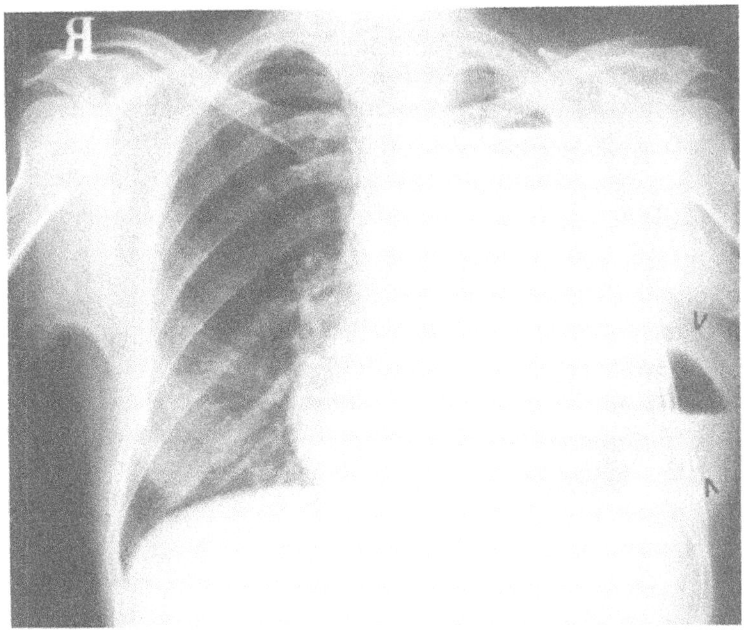

Fig. 17. Example of late empyema following a left pneumonectomy without stump leak (patient B. K., m., 54 years of age, pT3, N 1, M 0 squamous cell carcinoma, postoperative mediastinal radiation, 6 years' asymptomatic survial, died at 7 years from squamous cell carcinoma of light lung.) PA chest radiograph shows an apical fluid level on the left side where the lung was previously opaque. The second fluid level indicates empyema necessitans (*Staph. aureus*) of the extrathoracic soft tissues. Note the elevated diaphragm and the rounded gastric contour below. The empyema resolved after rethoracotomy and suction irrigation with chloramine

over next 12 months. Patient is asymptomatic almost 7 years after residual pneumonectomy and 5 years after resolution of empyema. Liver appeared normal at cholecystectomy in 1984.

As in the surgical treatment of bronchial stump leak, suction irrigation has proved its value in the management of postresection empyema, as three of four early infections and one late empyema resolved within 4 weeks or less. It is our impression that success can be achieved more quickly and reliably through irrigation with antiseptic solutions such as chloramine or Betadine than with local antibiotics (e.g., Polybactrin, Neomycin, Colistin). An important advantage, certainly, is the ability of irrigating solutions to deliver bactericidal agents to all sites within the pleural cavity, as Urfer et al. [343] have pointed out.

A potential cause of postresection empyema is intraoperative bacterial contamination, for, as mentioned earlier, pulmonary resections that open the major airways are not strictly aseptic procedures [188]. But early postoperative empyemas almost always occur in association with bronchopleural fistulas [22] or as a sequel to wound infection [32].

A third way in which pyothorax can arise is by blood-borne infection, which is believed to account for late empyema in the absence of a recurrent, perforating carcinoma of the stump [170]. Onsets as late as several years after pneumonectomy have been described [325].

Treatment consists of evacuation followed by closed drainage or suction irrigation, or open drainage through a thoracic window [170, 172, 343]. The latter always implies a chronic course. Definitive cure may be effected later with a thoracoplasty [342] if the empyema cavity does not obliterate spontaneously.

Complications of Postoperative Ventilation

With appropriate standards of postoperative patient care, ventilatory complications are rare. That they have not been entirely eliminated is illustrated by the case of a 60-year-old man who underwent a right upper lobectomy. A defect in the expiratory valve of the ventilator led to a massive increase in ventilatory pressure, which was only partly compensated by drainage on the operated side. The problem was not recognized until a tension pneumothorax had developed on the healthy side. The life-threatening complication was successfully managed by prompt decompressive drainage of the pneumothorax; there were no sequelae.

Chapter 5

Adjunctive Therapies

In a number of patients treatment was not limited to surgical resection, but was supplemented by preoperative or postoperative radiotherapy, cytostatic therapy, or their combination. Exploratory thoracotomies likewise were followed by the use of one or both alternative modalities. In some cases the surgical resection of metastatic cancers served an adjunctive goal.

Radiotherapy

A basic distinction is made between selective adjuvant therapy and the use of radiation for treatment of recurrent cancer.

Adjuvant Radiotherapy

Throughout the study there was interdisciplinary agreement concerning the use of adjuvant postoperative radiotherapy following 1) radical resections for mediastinal lymph node involvement, 2) extended resections for chest-wall and direct mediastinal invasion, and 3) peribronchial or submucous tumor spread in the area of bronchial transection at the trachea. The use of radiotherapy was contingent upon the patient's consent to the treatment and his presumed ability to tolerate it.

On that basis 38 patients were potential candidates for adjuvant postoperative radiotherapy, as shown in Table 31. Five of the patients were classified as operative mortalities, and six others refused postoperative radiation. In another five patients adjuvant radiotherapy was considered inappropriate because of age, general debilitation, or doubtful radiocurability. In four cases radiation had to be discontinued early because of progressive weakness.

Eighteen patients received a "curative" dose of 6000 rads. One of these patients is still alive eight years after surgery and radiotherapy. Four others survived between 5 and 10 years.

Among the patients with a T3 lesion who did not receive adjuvant radiotherapy, one patient who refused this therapy survived for 10 years. He died from pneumonia and right heart failure at 64 years of age. There was no clinical evidence of recurrence, and an autopsy was not performed.

Table 31

Patient, age, sex		Cell type	Radiotherapy	Course	Recurrence
Utilization of postoperative radiotherapy in N 2 cases					
1. B.T.,	43, f.	Adeno	Yes	†24 months	Yes
2. H.H.,	42, m.	Adeno	Yes	† 4.5 months	2nd carcinoma
3. J.R.,	67, m.	Squam	Yes	† 6 months	Yes (brain)
4. K.U.,	43, f.	Mucoep	Yes	† 8 months	Yes
5. M.E.,	48, m.	Squam	Yes	†26 months	Yes
6. M.K.,	56, m.	Squam	Yes	†24 months	Yes
7. S.M.,	65, m.	Squam	Yes	†51 months	No
8. G.A.,	65, m.	Squam	Yes	† 6.5 years	Yes
9. S.R.,	37, m.	Adeno	Yes	Surv. 8 yrs	No
10. B.K.,	70, m.	Squam	Refused	†13 months	Yes
11. G.G.,	53, m.	Squam	Refused	† 6 months	Unknown
12. T.B.,	48, m.	Small	Chemotherapy	†25 months	Yes
13–16 Operative mortality					
Utilization of postoperative radiotherapy for T3: Chest wall invasion					
1. R.M.,	56, m.	LCU	Yes	† 9 months	2nd carcinoma
2. M.E.,	72, m.	Squam	4000 rads	† 6 months	Yes (pulm. embolism)
3. S.R.,	54, m.	Adeno	Yes	† 8 months	Yes
4. S.J.,	69, m.	Squam	Yes		? (moved to Spain 8 months postop.)
5. R.H.,	72, f.	LCU	No (age/GC)	†24 months	Yes
6. H.R.,	54, m.	LCU	No (GC)	† 1.5 months	Yes
Utilization of postoperative radiotherapy for T3: Mediastinal invasion					
1. M.H.,	60, m.	Adeno	Yes	†30 months	No, 2nd carc.
2. M.W.,	51, m.	Squam	Yes	†16 months	Yes
3. S.J.,	50, m.	Squam	Yes	† 5.5 years	Yes, local
4. K.G.,	66, m.	Squam	Incomp. (GC)	† 3 months	No
5. B.A.,	73, m.	Squam	2000 rads (GC)	† 4.5 months	Yes
6. F.E.,	66, m.	Adeno	Refused	†30 months	Yes
7. G.A.,	63, m.	Squam	Refused	†38 months	Yes
8. J.W.,	54, m.	Squam	Refused	†10 years	No (autopsy)
9. K.K.,	68, f.	Adeno	No (GC)	†18 months	No, 2nd carc.
10. K.A.,	56, m.	Squam	Open T.b.	† 6 months	Yes
Utilization of postoperative radiotherapy for T3: Peribronchial tumor extension to within 1 cm of trachea					
1. B.K.,	54, m.	Squam	Yes	† 7 years	Yes
2. L.P.,	59, m.	Squam	Yes	† 5 months	? (†France)
3. M.J.,	60, m.	Squam	Yes	† 5 months	Yes
4. S.R.,	71, m.	Terato	No	† 6 months	Yes
5. Operative mortality					
6.[a] D.J.,	65, m.	Small/ squam	3000 rads postop.	† 4.5 years	Yes, brain metastasis (autopsy: no local recurrence)

[a] Preoperative treatment with 3000 rads for primarily inoperable tumor

Abbreviations:

Squam	Squamous cell carcinoma	Mucoep:	Mucoepidermoid carcinoma
Adeno:	Adenocarcinoma	GC:	General condition
Small:	Small cell carcinoma	†:	Died
LCU:	Large cell undiff. carcinoma		

According to Buenemann and Heilmann [44], radiation is capable of destroying squamous cell carcinomas and adenocarcinomas when delivered in an adequate dose (up to 8000 rads). This is confirmed for squamous cell carcinoma by Wannenmacher and Slanina [349]. A number of other authors express basically the same view [191, 284]. Radiotherapy with curative intent has been advocated by many as an alternative to surgical resection, following the same criteria for local tumor extent, in patients who are inoperable for medical reasons or who will not submit to surgery [6, 85, 133, 134, 158]. However, the 5-year survival rates for such cases, at 8%–22% in early-stage cancers [44, 191], are markedly lower than when radiotherapy is preceded by resection.

Thus, from the standpoint of the thoracic surgeon who must be content with a questionably curative resection or, for technical reasons, a resection that is frankly incomplete, the postoperative irradiation of suspected or confirmed residual tumor is a logical measure for improving the therapeutic outcome [187]. Whereas Matthews et al. [212] are skeptical as to the benefits of postoperative radiation, Kirsh et al. [173] report 5-year survival rates as high as 40% in squamous cell carcinoma and 18% in adenocarcinoma with postoperative irradiation of mediastinal metastases. No patient who did not receive radiotherapy was a 5-year survivor. In a study by Gobbel et al. [94], radiotherapy following incomplete lung cancer resections caused a flattening of the mortality curve in the first 2 years after surgery, although there were still no 5-year survivors. In a group of patients who had had curative resections, postoperative radiotherapy had no discernible effect on long-term survival.

On the other hand, Choi [51 a] and other authors have observed that adjuvant radiotherapy with curative intent markedly improves actuarial survival rates in N 1 and N 2 cases as well as in patients with T 3 cancers. However, Choi also stresses the importance of selecting patients on the basis of pulmonary function criteria (FEV_1 at least 1.25 L or 45% normal, VC at least 1.75 L or 45% normal, P_aO_2 at least 70 mm Hg).

There is a lack of controlled, randomized studies on this question. Cohen [56] reports that the Working Party for Lung Cancer (WP-L) is presently conducting studies on the effect of radiotherapy as an adjunct to complete and incomplete resections of stage III squamous cell carcinomas of the lung.

Our own results are insufficient to support one opinion over the other because of our limited case numbers and because of the positive selection effect of withholding postoperative radiotherapy from patients whose general condition was poor as a result of their tumor or other causes. Episodic evidence of favorable responses to postoperative radiotherapy and the proven fact that radiation can be destructive to bronchogenic carcinoma justify maintaining, at least for the present, the indications for adjuvant radiotherapy stated above.

Radiotherapy of Metastatic and Recurrent Disease

In 15 patients, *local recurrences* prompted the use of radiotherapy at varying intervals after surgery (up to 5 years). The most common immediate indications were massive hemoptysis (9 cases), atelectasis (3 cases), and chest wall pain (3 cases).

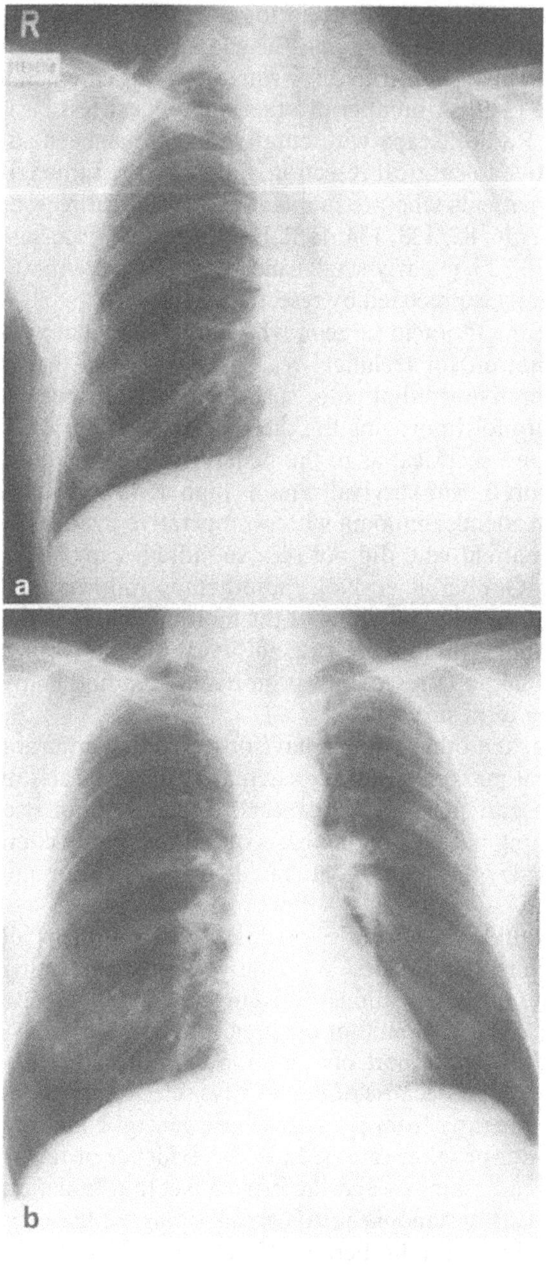

Fig. 18. a Example of preoperative radiotherapy of lung carcinoma. PA chest radiograph (patient D. J., m., 65 years of age, pT3, N1, M0 squamous cell carcinoma of left main bronchus). There is total atelectasis of the left lung from complete obstruction of the main bronchus, with a marked leftward shift of the mediastinum. **b** Same patient: radiographic appearance after 3000 rads with the left lung reventilated and a now visible central mass. (After pneumonectomy and complementary 3000 rads no local recurrence 4 years later at death, caused by exclusively cerebral spread.)

Bone metastases in five patients were irradiated for relief of pain, and brain metastases were irradiated in two others. In all cases the malignant process was no longer curable. The radiation dose did not exceed 3800 rads. The therapy, which in some cases was combined with chemotherapy, relieved certain distressing symptoms but presumably did not produce a significant increase in survival.

Preoperative Radiotherapy

A program for the use of adjuvant preoperative radiotherapy did not exist in the present series. Nevertheless, the combination of preoperative radiotherapy and surgial resection happened to occur in two of our male patients.

1. M. W., 56 years of age: In 1973 the patient was diagnosed elsewhere as having an undifferentiated carcinoma in the left main bronchus. There was concomitant fever and pleural effusion without cells. Inoperability was assumed, and 6000 rads of radiation was administered. Later surgery was considered because of residual tumor with a radiographic density in the left lower lung. Pneumonectomy was done 3 weeks after discontinuance of radiotherapy and 4 months after diagnosis, revealing a central, poorly differentiated squamous cell carcinoma without lymph node metastases that had invaded the central pulmonary vessels. The postoperative course was uneventful. Patient is surving 11½ years and worked half days until his retirement.
2. D. J., 65 years of age (Fig. 18): Total atelectasis of the left lung secondary to *small cell anaplastic* carcinoma of the main bronchus closely approaching the bifurcation. Primary surgery was rejected on technical and histologic grounds. Irradiation with 3000 rads caused marked regression of the tumor, and surgery was reconsidered. With negative mediastinoscopy, a left pneumonectomy was performed 3 weeks after discontinuance of radiotherapy. Recovery was uneventful except for atrial fibrillation. Histology showed poorly differentiated *squamous cell carcinoma* with adenomatous elements. The intra- and interlobar lymph nodes were involved by tumor, prompting saturation with an additional 3000 rads. Brain metastases appeared 30 months later, prompting surgery and postoperative radiation, probably not curative. The patient survived almost 5 years. Autopsy confirmed brain metastases but showed no thoracic recurrence.

The preoperative irradiation of inoperable or marginally inoperable tumors has frequently been recommended. In relating his experience with preoperative radiation, Viereck [344] states that after a dose of 6000 rads is delivered, surgical resection is no longer possible because of the extreme difficulty of isolating the hilar structures. We personally had no problems of this nature in the case described above. Preoperative radiation is acknowledged to have value in the management of "Pancoast's tumors" [19, 109, 253]. However, Cohen [56] states that routine preoperative radiotherapy has not proved beneficial, and Harmon et al. [113] and Johnson [158] call attention to the possibility of an increased rate of postoperative complications.

Adjunctive Chemotherapy

In contrast to radiotherapy, which was used as an adjuvant in certain situations, cytostatic therapy after cancer surgery was limited to patients with tumor progression and to an additional 10 patients who had undergone exploratory thoracotomies.

Only one patient with squamous cell carcinoma was treated preoperatively with a four-drug combination (cyclophosphamide, procarbazin, vincristine, methotrexate) and was referred eight months after diagnosis with total atelectasis of the left lung that developed during therapy. The operation had to be concluded as an exploratory thoracotomy, and so no effect on surgical outcome can be discerned.

The same combination therapy was given to four patients whose surgery at stage I was followed by recurrence and metastasis of large cell undifferentiated carcinoma (2) and squamous cell carcinoma (2) after local irradiation. Three patients survived 2–3 months after the initiation of chemotherapy for recurrent cancer, and 1 survived 9 months.

One patjent who had undergone surgery for squamous cell carcinoma developed a small cell carcinoma of the opposite side one year postoperatively and survived another seven months on chemotherapy.

Chemotherapy was also given to 7 patients who had been operated on for stage III cancers (4 adenocarcinomas, 1 large cell carcinoma, 1 small cell carcinoma, 1 undifferentiated squamous cell carcinoma). The longest survival time, 24 months, was in a young woman who had undergone a palliative adjuvant lobectomy with lymphadenectomy followed by radiation and continued chemotherapy (see Fig. 10).

It must be concluded that chemotherapy in this series did not improve five-year survival rates and indeed had no effect on survival beyond two years.

The ability of systematic adjuvant chemotherapy to improve surgical results [130, 168, 358, 365] remains questionable. A worsening of results, meanwhile, has been observed and reported by various authors [56, 65, 310].

Adjuvant Immunotherapy

During the final year of this study 23 patients were enrolled in a comparative prospective study (European Multicenter Trial) on the possible benefits of *Corynebacterium parvum* administered intrapleurally after lung cancer surgery [197a]. Subsequent evaluation has failed to demonstrate a beneficial effect in the 10 patients who received the bacterium. Selection criteria were age under 70 years and the presence of a stage I or stage II non-small cell cancer. We found identical survival rates and failure rates in both the treated group and the controls. Today, more than 6 years later, 11 of the 23 patients are still alive, and 3 others survived longer than 5 years.

Surgical Treatment of Brain Metastases

Adjunctive therapies included *surgical interventions* for metastatic disease. All of these involved the resection of solitary brain metastases, combined in some cases with postoperative radiation.

The decision to operate for brain metastasis is easily made when the metastatic lesion is favorably located, the general condition of the patient is still good, and no other demonstrable metastases are present.

Table 32. Resections of brain metastases

Patient, age, sex	Stage/ cell type	Interval since lung operation	Course	Interval since brain operation	Total survival	Autopsy findings
A.N., 57, m.	I, LCU	56 months	Died	2 weeks	56 months	Pulmonary embolism, no distant metast.
B.W., 58, m.	II, Squam	17 months/ 19 months	Died	8/6 months	25 months	No autopsy
H.S., 66, m.	I, Squam	18 months	Died	24 months	42 months	Recurrence of brain metast. only
R.K., 39, m.	I, Squam	18 months	Died	10 months	28 months	No autopsy
E.H., 58, m.	III, LCU	9 months	Died	48 months	69 months	No autopsy
D.J., 65, m.	III, Squam	26 months	Died	20 months	58 months	Recurrence of brain metast. only

LCU: Large cell undiff. carcinoma
Squam: Squamous cell carcinoma

In addition, the clinical situation often justifies intervention even if conditions are relatively unfavorable and the risk is relatively high.

Six patients in this series underwent resections of brain metastases. One patient was operated on twice. The results with respect to survival times appear more favorable than in cases where metastases and recurrences in general were treated with radiation and drugs (Table 32). One patient survived longer than five years, and one died shortly before five years from a pulmonary embolism following resection of his brain metastasis.

It is noteworthy that autopsy in three cases showed no metastases occurring outside the brain – an observation which strengthens the justification for a more aggressive approach to cerebral metastases.

Chapter 6

Aftercare

The organization of a systematic program of aftercare was consistent with the prospective concept of our study. However, certain difficulties arose and are continuing to arise due to the negative attitude of some private practitioners, who either regard centralized aftercare as a form of competition or feel that their competence is being questioned. Nevertheless, we were successful for the most part in alerting private physicians to the importance of the continuing care of patients who have undergone cancer surgery. The patients are virtually unanimous in their assent to the continuation of surgical care beyond the operation itself, and in fact many show an attitude of outright insistence, as may be inferred from the spontaneous inquiries that are received when a scheduled examination is delayed.

Scheduling of Follow-Up Visits

We examined the patients at three-month intervals for the first three years after surgery. We have been able to confirm that, regardless of tumor stage and histology, a marked flattening of the survival curve occurs after the third postoperative year. In the 4th and 5th years examinations are scheduled at 6-month intervals, and then at 12-month intervals thereafter.

Simple Examination

With passage of time we simplified the procedure for follow-up examinations. The core of the examination is an interview in which the patient is asked about his intervening history, his tolerance for exercise, and his subjective sense of well-being. A physical examination is made of the thoracic organs and upper-body lymph nodes, and the patient is weighed.

In the absence of specific indications, we no longer order routine blood studies. The only special investigation is the obtaining of chest radiographs in two planes, which we read in the presence of the patient.

Constancy of Personnel

We feel it is essential that the patient always be confronted with "his own" physician if at all possible. This is not only helpful psychologically, but it enhances the value of the examination and makes it possible to dispense with unnecessary tests. The follow-up examination, then, should be conducted either by the physician who performed the operation or by a physician who has known and followed the patient for some time.

Communication with the Family Physician

The aftercare facility cannot and should not usurp the role of the family physician [239]. Any resentment that is directed toward centralized aftercare by specialists is often rooted in an inadequate exchange of information. We made it a practice, therefore, to report findings to private physicians and include recommendations for any additional tests that we felt were necessary.

Assessment of Disability

It is not unusual for patients with a physically demanding occupation to find that, at some point in their postoperative course, they are no longer able to meet accustomed job demands [141, 179]. Usually these are patients who have already survived several years after their operation, and in whom the summation of age- and surgery-related functional limitations is creating a state of incipient decompensation. In such cases the aftercare facility plays an important role in the evaluation of patients who make application for partial disability or early retirement.

What initially had been planned as a critical study of the surgical treatment of lung carcinoma very soon developed into an institution whose main function was the serving of patient needs. The therapeutic options in the face of recurrent cancer are generally very limited. Nevertheless, in many cases symptoms could be ameliorated or relieved by the verification of bone metastases, for example, and the early initiation of palliative radiotherapy. In a few cases secondary operations were performed after new pulmonary tumors were diagnosed. More frequently, measures were instituted for treatment of functional decompensation, including chronic broncholytic therapy, digitalization, conversion of disabling intercurrent atrial fibrillation, and even operative treatment for progressive mitral insufficiency. It is not uncommon for patients to turn to the aftercare facility when their personal physician is unavailable, thus emphasizing the nature of the services provided. Valuable experience is gained in many areas of operative management such as the prophylaxis and reduction of chronic thoracotomy-related complaints, and in the selection of patients for procedures such as palliative resections and reoperations. The lack of an aftercare program would create a serious information gap that would leave many detailed questions unanswered.

Ninety-five percent of all patients have been and are being managed by a centralized aftercare facility, some over long distances. A few patients have refused aftercare either on their own initiative or on the advice of their physician. In a small number, regular pneumologic examinations are performed in outlying offices and the results are forwarded to a central facility.

To monitor survival in patients not enrolled in our aftercare program, we elicited the support of the tumor registry serving the city of Basel and the surrounding district. For patients living outside that district, we directed necessary inquiries to family physicians or relatives.

Problems of Aftercare

In a decentralized health-care system, aftercare is associated with a number of essentially organizational problems. The necessity of aftercare for the critical evaluation of operative therapy is not disputed. The responsibility, therefore, belongs in the hands of the surgeon [178].

One function of oncologic aftercare is to document the postoperative course of a surgically treated cancer patient for an indefinitive period or until death occurs. Thus, it is necessary not only to record the time and cause of death, but also to determine whether and what type of chronic complaints were present and how the patient's quality of life was affected.

Equal in importance to observation and documentation are measures directed toward the treatment of any side effects and sequelae that may arise [359]. This includes the recognition and treatment of impending right heart failure after pneumonectomy [233] as well as the early detection of recurrent cancer and the assessment of its resectability.

In theory these functions could be accomplished without centralized aftercare, but practice has shown that effective supervision is very difficult to maintain when such an organization does not exist. Patients who believe that they have been cured by their operation and are free of symptoms often suppress the memory of their illness and do not present for examinations unless they are summoned.

Follow-up, an essential part of aftercare, is practiced with varying degrees of success. Overholt et al. [249] lost only 1.3% of their patients to follow-up in more than 1800 resections in 42 years. Belcher and Anderson [21] lost 1%, and Taylor [332] lost 0.1%. On the other hand, there are publications that must limit reports on long-term results to only a portion of the primary population. In many of these studies, additional information would have to be sought from patients, relatives, physicians, and public agencies in order to make the results meaningful. Hoffmann et al. [136] followed 70% of patients operated at the Dusseldorf University Clinic, and Guetgemann et al. [103] followed 85% of surgical patients at the Bonn Clinic. An equal follow-up rate is reported by Baldamus and Ceh [15]. Many authors ignore the question of the completeness of postoperative follow-up.

In a major collaborative study conducted in the Federal Republic of Germany [20], course data were available for 68% of 3500 patients operated on before 1969. The authors' calculations of 5 year survival rates for the principal cancer cell types resected at stage T1/T2, N0, M0 are based on a total of only 164 observations. Studies like this one support the statement made by Trendelenburg in 1977 [338] and repeated by Barth in 1981 [17] that controlled prospective studies on surgical therapy are rare.

We must admit, however, that our own follow-up program profitted from two favorable circumstances. First, our frequency of operations was low compared with large thoracic surgical centers, and second, the geographic area served by our clinic was relatively small.

Chapter 7

Results

Operative Mortality

The early deaths that followed exploratory thoracotomies and tumor resections were mentioned previously in connection with complications. Here we shall present a general overview of the operative deaths (30 days) and hospital deaths that occurred in this series. Early mortality not only influences the definitive survival results, but also is a criterion that is much more salient than long- term results and thus has a very strong impact on the reputation of surgical resection as a treatment method.

The 12 cases of operative and hospital mortality are listed chronologically in Table 33.

Table 33. Operative (30-day) mortality and hospital mortality

Year	Patient	Age	Tumor stage	Operation	Complications	Interval to operation
1972	S.W., m.	69	III	Pneumonectomy	Pulm. embolism	9 days
1972	R.D., m.	59	III	Pneumonectomy	Pulm. embolism	2 days
1973	W.K., m.	61	III	Lobectomy	Pulm. embolism	4 days
1973	K.R., m.	56	III	Rad. pneumect.	Cerebromalacia, second. pneumonia	6 days
1973	B.R., m.	66	III	Rad. pneumect.	Stump leak, pneumonia	9 days
1973	M.F., m.	63	III	Thoracotomy	Intraoperative bleeding	–
1973	G.K., m.	66	I	Sleeve lobect.	Cerebrovascular accident, secondary pneumonia	35 days
1974	J.T., m.	60	III	Thoracotomy	Cerebrovascular accident with brain metastases	23 days
1974	E.B., m.	69	I	Lobectomy	Gastric bleeding, after 2nd laparotomy pulm. embolism	32 days
1975	B.A., m.	64	III	Rad. pneumect.	Pulm. embolism	2 days
1975	K.H., m.	48	III	Rad. lobect.	Acute cardiac death with aortic stenosis	8 hours
1976	S.J., m.	65	I	Lobectomy	Intestinal compl.†op., second. pneumonia	7 days

As we saw in Fig. 2, half of all perioperative deaths occurred in the years 1972 and 1973. The leading cause was fulminant pulmonary embolism, which accounted for 50% of fatalities.

We also find that 9 early deaths occurred in patients with an advanced stage III tumor, equaling a 17% mortality rate (9 of 52). Because a relatively large percentage of operations in this group were pneumonectomies, we find a correspondingly higher mortality for this type of resection. Thirty-day mortality included 5 deaths in 72 pneumonectomies, for a rate of 7%, and 3 deaths in 122 lobectomies, for a rate of only 2.5%. The hospital mortality for lobectomies and bilobectomies (including secondary operations) was 4%.

As the frequency of operations increased in the period from 1974 to 1978, the mortality rate declined. Apparently this is based not on a lower incidence of technical problems, but on more efficient postoperative management procedures, especially with regard to the shortening and simplification of postoperative intensive care and earlier ambulation.

We investigated other factors that might affect the incidence of postoperative deaths. Thus, we noted that the proportion of pneumonectomies to lobectomies in 1972, at 1.0, was higher than in subsequent years, while the figure of 0.7 in 1973 was exactly equal to that in 1977 and 1978.

We found no differences with regard to age distribution or preoperative defects of cardiorespiratory function. Indeed, as the study progressed we elected surgery more frequently in patients whose functional operability was marginal.

Two deaths occurred in connection with exploratory thoracotomies performed in patients with inoperable cancer. One death resulted from intraoperative hemorrhage, and the other occurred at 3 weeks from cerebral complications precipitated by a previously undiagnosed brain metastasis. This corresponds to an 11% mortality rate for exploratory thoracotomy without resection, an indication that this procedure should be avoided if at all possible [18].

Long-Term Results

Method of Evaluation

It is customary to measure the efficacy of cancer surgery by the actual or probable duration and frequency of survival. In the present study we are not concerned with comparing different methods of patient selection or treatment, because, with the exception of a few modifications made in evaluation procedures, we applied uniform guidelines to the selection and operation of all 206 patients over a period of almost 7 years. Experience gained during the course of the study mainly influenced postoperative management and, with it, the perioperative mortality discussed in the previous section.

The following variables, then, can be tested with regard to their effect on postoperative survival: tumor stage, tumor histology, the extent of surgery, and the general condition of the patient.

Survival calculations are limited to patients whose tumors were surgically resectable; 18 exploratory thoracotomies without resection are disregarded. No attempt is made to correlate survival with sex, because the number of female patients is too small to provide meaningful data.

As stated earlier, patients who were not available for follow-up were excluded from evaluation, thereby eliminating the speculative factor of incomplete observations [71]. We were able to maintain continual follow-up in 187 consecutive patients.

Our study is incomplete only with respect to the duration of follow-up. This is characteristic of all clinical investigations that employ an essentially unlimited period of follow-up and analyze results without awaiting the deaths of all patients. Methods of drawing valid conclusions from incomplete observations were developed by Cutler and Ederer [59] and Kaplan and Meier [165] and are widely utilized.

Our data were processed using the University of California Biomedical Data Program for calculating life tables and survival functions [268]. The end point for the input of survival data was February 28, 1985. The first resection was performed on February 11, 1972, and the last on August 28, 1978. The longest period of follow-up was 13 years, the shortest 6.5 years.

Overview (Table 34)

Forty-six of 187 patients who underwent cancer resections are still alive. Seventy-four patients have survived longer than five years, or had survived that long at the time of their deaths.

The 5-year cumulative survival rate for all patients who underwent resective surgery, independent of tumor stage and histology, is 39.5% (S.E. ± 3.6%). Since our initial calculation 5 years ago (12-31-79) this figure has declined by 3.3%.

Effect of Tumor Stage (Fig. 19a)

Thirty-one of 91 patients with stage I tumors are still alive. The maximum survival to date is 12.7 years. The 5-year survival rate is 53.8% (S.E. ± 5.3%).

We find that the percentages are significantly smaller for patients with stage II and stage III disease. Thus, only 11 of 53 patients with stage III cancer survived longer than 5 years.

Effect of Tumor Histology (Fig. 19b)

We could find no statistically significant differences between squamous cell carcinoma and adenocarcinoma, which accounted for the majority of lung can-

Table 34. Summary of statistical results of survival

	Patients (n)	Death (n)	Surv. (n)	Mean surv. (days)	S.E. (days)	Median surv. (days)	Cumulative survival rates %				Sig.
							1 year	3 yrs.	5 yrs.	10 yrs.	
Total	187	141	46	1758	125	945	74.3	46.5	39.5	22.8	
Stage I	91	60	31	2238	186	2285	83.5	60.4	53.8	28.8	
Stage II	43	32	11	1710	251	883	83.7	41.8	34.9	24.2	$p<0.001$
Stage III	53	49	4	914	161	402	52.8	26.4	18.9	4.7	
Histology											
Squamous cell	124	93	31	1801	156	1076	72.6	49.2	41.1	21.7	$p<0.5$
Adeno	40	29	11	1723	236	945	85.0	42.5	42.5	21.2	n.s.
Large cell/other	19	15	4	1153	253	732	68.4	42.1	26.3	21.0	
Small cell	4	4	0	864	503	706	75.0	25.0	25.0	–	
Type of resection											
Lobectomy	118	88	30	1783	160	945	77.0	44.9	39.8	22.8	$p<0.6$
Pneumonectomy	69	53	16	1685	195	895	71.0	49.0	39.0	17.5	n.s.

cers. The cumulative 5-year survival rates for these tumors are 41.1% and 42.5%, respectively. Our statistical results for the group of predominantly large cell undifferentiated carcinomas and for the very small number of small cell undifferentiated cancers are of little significance. Of four patients in the latter group whose cancers were technically resectable, only one survived for six years.

Effect of Extent of Resection (Fig. 19c)

We also wished to determine whether the type of operation performed – lobectomy or pneumonectomy – had an impact on survival rates, since the decision between these operations has several, partially conflicting aspects. On the one hand, the more extensive the operation, the greater the chance for eliminating the tumor. On the other hand, more extensive resections in our series were usually associated with more extensive tumor involvement, and also with more severe losses of function.

A comparison of the mortality curves after pneumonectomy vs. lobectomy, however, shows no obvious differences aside from the operative mortality, which determines the initial shape of the curve. With passage of time, deaths of lobectomized patients become predominant because of their greater primary incidence. The cumulative survival rate at the end of 5 years is 40% for both types of resection. Only after 10 years the cumulative survival rate of patients after pneumonectomy compared to those after lobectomy tends to drop slightly (17.5% vs. 22.8%); however, this difference does not reach statistical significance.

Effect of Age

By now it is apparent that the tumor stage has by far the greatest impact on life expectancy. We sought to determine what effect, if any, the patient's chronologic age had on the postoperative course. We therefore made a comparison between patients 60 years of age or older ($n = 107$) and patients under 60 years of age ($n = 80$). The cumulative survival rate at the end of 5 years was 37% in the older group, as opposed to 44% in the younger group. However, statistical significance could not be demonstrated when the factor of tumor stage was taken into account ($p = 0.25$).

Effect of Delay Time

To obtain groups of sufficient size, we divided the patients into groups with delay times less than 100 days and delay times greater than 100 days (about 3 months). We then checked for correlation with survival. While we had expected that survival would correlate inversely with delay in surgery, this could not be confirmed. We did note that mortality in the first postoperative year was higher

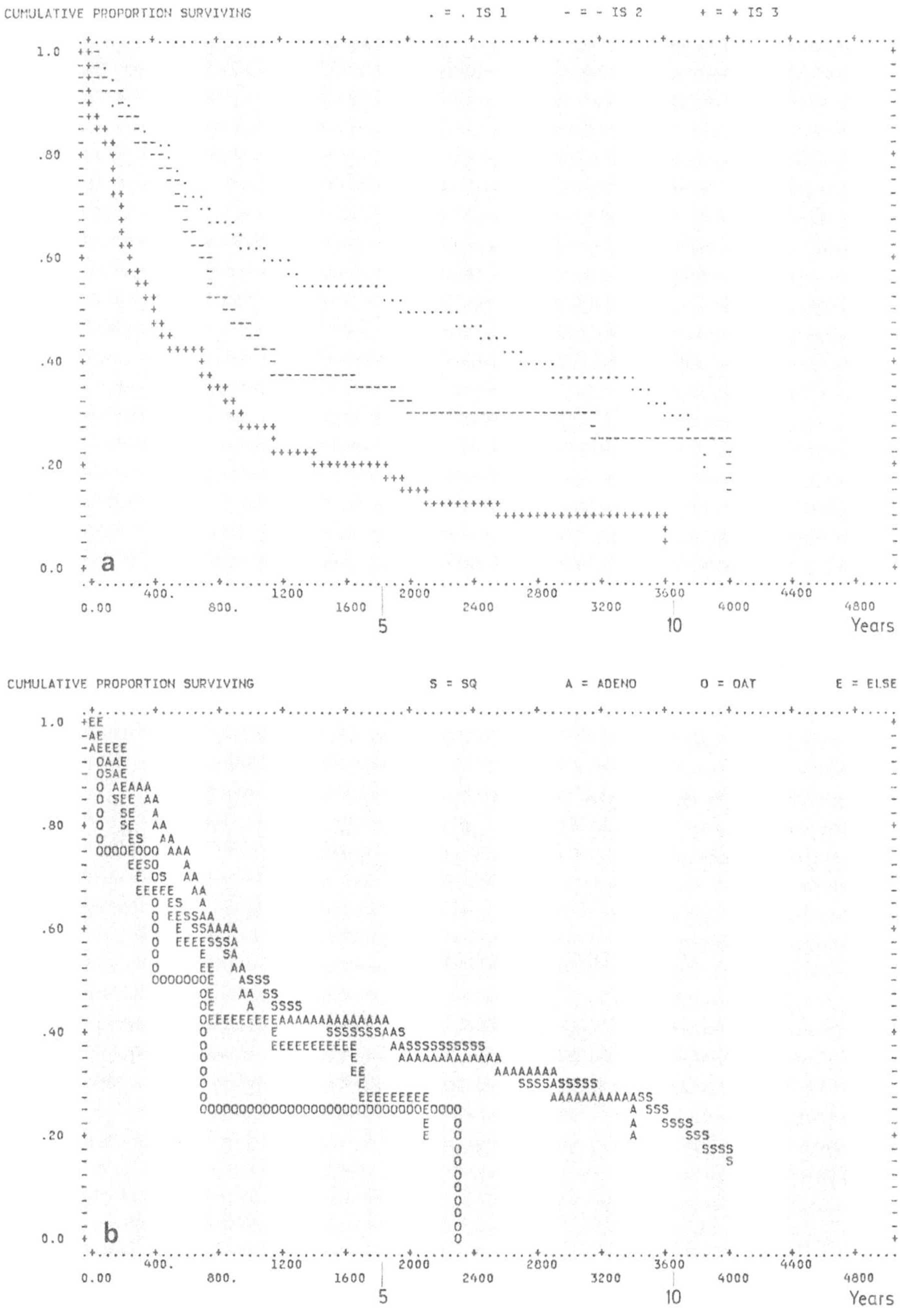

Fig. 19. a Cumulative survival rates by pTNM stage. ....=Stage I. ---=Stage II. +++=Stage III. **b** Cumulative survival rates by *tumor histology*. S=squamous cell carcinoma; A=adenocarcinoma; O=small cell undifferentiated carcinoma; E=large cell and other carcinomas. No difference is apparent between squamous cell carcinoma and adenocarcinoma. Statistically valid data are not available for the remaining groups

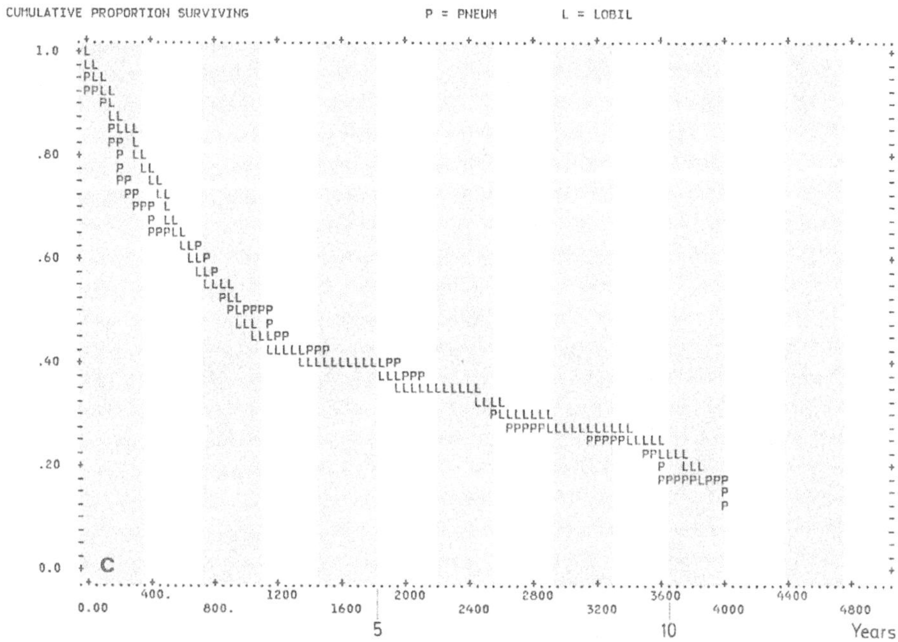

Fig. 19. c Cumulative survival rates by *type of resection*. P = pneumonectomy; L = lobectomy/bilobectomy

in the group with the greater delay (30% vs. 21.6%), but the difference was not significant. After the second postoperative year, mortality in the group with the greater delay time was lower both relatively and absolutely.

Effect of Cardiorespiratory Function

Working from the premise that adverse effects of diminished cardiorespiratory function on immediate and long-term results would be most apparent in patients with severe dysfunctions, we investigated the fates of the function-impaired groups.

Of the 15 patients with *active pulmonary artery hypertension* (Table 21), who had varying degrees of coexisting obstructive lung disease, 1 patient died 2 days after pneumonectomy with the clinical diagnosis of pulmonary embolism. Of the remaining 3 pneumonectomized patients, 2 survived for 7 months and 40 months; 1 patient (stage I small cell carcinoma, residual pneumonectomy after previous resection for bronchiectasis) survived 6 years, had returned to work, experienced dyspnea only with moderately severe to severe exertion, and was active recreationally to a limited degree. Ten patients in this group underwent lobectomies. One of these, a 54-year-old man, died at 51 days from what was presumed to be a progression of his lung cancer. He had the highest pulmonary arterial resistance measured in this group: 5.3 units. Autopsy was not performed. The impression of bronchial carcinoma as the cause of death appears to be justified by the incomplete, secondary palliative resection of large cell carcinoma with chest-wall invasion that had been performed in this patient. Of the remaining patients, four died from recurrent cancer, one died from an autonomous brain tumor (sarcoma), and one died from clinically diagnosed heart failure. Three patients survived between 45 and 85 months. There was only one instance, therefore, where pulmonary artery hypertension appeared to correlate with decreased survival.

Another group of patients had a predominantly *respiratory* function impairment (see Table 22). This group included 19 patients with severe bronchopulmonary obstruction, 3 with severe restrictive ventilatory impairment, and 5 with a combination of both. Eleven of the patients had a coexisting diffusion defect.

None of these 27 patients died in connection with their operation, though it should be noted that most underwent partial resections, which carry a lower primary mortality. While the proportion of lobectomies to pneumonectomies in the overall series was 1.7 (122:72), it was 3.5 (21:6) in this group.

On the other hand, the prevalence of the different tumor stages in this group was similar to that in the series as a whole (15 patients stage I, 3 patients stage II, 9 patients stage III).

Of the five patients who are still alive, four experience dyspnea with moderate exertion, and one with mild exertion. Fourteen patients died from a recurrence or progression of their primary cancer, and 3 patients died from a coexisting, independent malignant disease. One patient died 9 months postoperatively at the age of 49 from cardiac failure, and another died 6 years after surgery from pneumonia and cardiac failure. Cause of death in the remaining patients is indefinite. One patient with a significant restrictive defect required continuous hospitalization and ventilatory assistance before dying from an extensive recurrence. This was the patient discussed previously who had surgery for recurrent cancer and underwent a tertiary residual pneumonectomy due to kinking of the bronchus (see p. 72).

Results of Resections in Patients over 70 Years of Age

Nineteen patients were in their eighth decade of life at operation. The average age of this group was 72.1 years. The following operations were performed:

Exploratory thoracotomy	1
Left pneumonectomy	3
Right pneumonectomy	1
Bilobectomy	3
Lobectomy	10
Lobectomy + chest wall resection	1

The patients were selected for operation using the same functional criteria that were applied to all patients. Only four were selected for pneumonectomy. All patients survived the surgery. Four patients reached or passed the 5-year mark, and 1 reached the age of 80 years. One man had to have an operation for a second carcinoma at the age of 76, 6 years after the first resection was performed. He has survived this operation more than three years with complete independence and moderate dyspnea.

Given the physiologic regression of functional reserves that occurs with age, pulmonary resection, especially pneumonectomy, is considered a difficult operation in patients over 70 years of age. The operative mortality in this age group is quite high. Jones et al. [160] indicate a primary mortality of 8.6% in a series of 35 elderly patients. Only 18 underwent lung resections, including 9 pneumonectomies, while 19 patients were explored without resection. All three deaths in this series occurred after pneumonectomies. Weiss [355] reports a mortality rate of 18.3% in 60 patients, which markedly exceeds the percentage of 5-year survivors. Hogsbro and Ostergard [137] report an operative mortality of 44% after pneumonectomy and 20% after lobectomy. In a study by Harviel et al. [116] in 32 patients over 70 years of age, 5 patients died within 30 days of lung cancer surgery – 4 who underwent resection and 1 of 10 who underwent exploratory thoracotomy (18%). In a retrospective study of 433 lung resections by Freise et al. [86], we find only 6 patients over 70 years of age (1.4%), none of whom was a 5-year survivor. Ross [278] writes in *Geriatrics* [1976] that "few patients over 65 or 70 years of age will tolerate a resection, especially if a pneumonectomy is required." This is in clear contradiction with our experience.

Results of Secondary Operations

Surgical reintervention for a new or recurrent cancer may be considered a priori only if the extent of the primary operation was limited to a lobectomy or bilobectomy. Another prerequisite is that the new tumor be removable by a contralateral partial resection or an ipsilateral residual pneumonectomy. Of course, the patient must be functionally able to tolerate the proposed resection.

A somewhat more difficult question is when a reoperation is reasonable from an oncologic standpoint. In the face of a local recurrence without demonstrable metastasis or a new primary tumor with a different histology, we feel that reoperation is justified. However, if a new tumor of identical histology is judged to be a product of hematogenous spread, then a major contraindication to surgical intervention would exist. This problem has been previously addressed by Boucot et al. [33] and by Merrick et al. [219].

Eleven patients in our series underwent secondary operations. This corresponds to 5.3% of all patients who had resective surgery. In three cases reintervention was motivated by local recurrences, in two cases by synchronous tumors, and in six cases by metachronous tumors. In all patients the histologies of the primary and secondary operations were identical. The interval between the two operations ranged from 4 days to 15 years.

Reintervention for Local Recurrence

All three affected patients had had their primary operations outside our clinic from seven weeks to three years previously.

1. F. M., 63 years of age, m.: Left lower lobectomy for squamous cell carcinoma. Incomplete resection, postoperative radiotherapy. Hemoptysis with bronchoscopically and histologically confirmed stump recurrence. Reoperated at 18 months. Died intraoperatively from aortic rupture (see p. 86).
2. S. A., 64 years of age, f. (Fig. 20): Segmentectomy for squamous cell carcinoma of the apex of the right upper lobe. Worsening of cough noted 2 years postoperatively. New density found in right upper lung, positive sputum cytology. Three years after primary operation, right pneumonectomy was performed for cancer spread to lower lobe. Patient has survived more than 8 years with grade III dyspnea and no signs of recurrence.
3. W. K., 58 years of age, m.: Segmentectomy for squamous cell carcinoma of the apex of the right upper lobe. Histologic examination of specimen showed line of resection crossing the tumor. Seven weeks later secondary resection of residual upper lobe and segment 6, which was integrated into the residual lobe. Specimen showed chronic inflammatory changes but no evidence of tumor. Residual pneumonectomy was done 4 weeks later because of recurrent sputum retention with bronchial collapse and kinking. Patient survived 11 months with grade III–IV respiratory failure and died from tumor recurrence (indurated mass in right chest cavity) and cardiac failure associated with coronary stenosis and multiple infarctions (see p. 72).

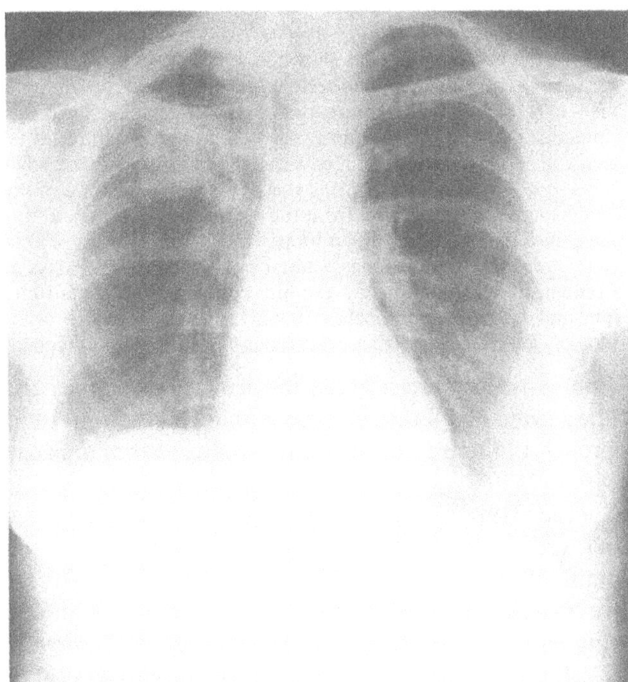

Fig. 20. Radiograph illustrating a local recurrence. Patient S. A., f., 63 years of age: squamous cell carcinoma, treated by S 1/2 segmentectomy performed elsewhere 33 months previously. At reoperation (pneumonectomy) the middle lobe and S6 were found to be invaded by tumor (pT2, N0, M0). Patient has survived > 8 years without recurrence

With one intraoperative death and one protracted course marked by respiratory failure and other serious problems, the results of these three reinterventions are not encouraging. Cases 1 and 3 document the importance of intraoperative frozen section examinations of resected specimens to confirm adequate margins. Cases 2 and 3 support our belief that an adequate carcinoma resection requires at least a lobectomy, though it must be acknowledged that favorable results have been achieved with lesser operations [180, 317, 364].

Synchronous Tumors

With synchronous lung tumors of identical histologies, it is impossible to tell with certainty whether both tumors are primary or whether one is primary and the other metastatic. For that reason the decision to operate is largely a matter of personal judgment. During staging we assumed we were dealing with a primary tumor and a metastasis (stage III disease) if the lesions were bilateral or if they occurred in two different lobes of the same lung. Nevertheless, we elected to perform surgical resection in two patients who had this pattern of disease.

1. B. W., 65 years of age, m. (Fig. 21): Lobectomy for peripheral squamous cell carcinoma of the right upper lobe without lymph node involvement. In 6th week of convalescence radiographs showed 2-cm density in left lower lobe. Follow-up showed marked enlargement of the mass, which was encroaching on the chest wall.
   The patient's functional status was good (static and dynamic volumes equaled the predicted), and a 2nd operation was performed 6 months after the first. In the 8 years since the 2nd operation the patient has shown no evidence of recurrence.
2. W. K., 61 years of age, m.: Lobectomy for peripheral squamous cell carcinoma in apical segment of left lower lobe. Preoperative diagnostic work-up was done elsewhere. Bronchoscopy immediately before thoracotomy showed no abnormalities in left lower lobe, but compression and subtle mucosal changes were noted at the segmental division of the left upper lobar bronchus. The upper lobar hilus was explored at the time of lower lobectomy, and a small hamartoma was enucleated from the segmental trifurcation. Bronchoscopy was repeated at the end of the operation, and a biopsy was taken. Histologic examination showed squamous cell carcinoma, prompting a residual pneumonectomy 4 days after the primary operation. Comparative histopathologic examination showed a 3-cm tumor in the apex of the lower lobe and a 5-mm endobronchial tumor in the upper lobe – both poorly differentiated squamous cell carcinomas. Patient is surviving 8 years without recurrence.

Both patients were selected for primary resective surgery without knowledge of the second neoplasm. The favorable results seem to justify a more aggressive approach to the treatment of multicentric carcinomas as has traditionally been advised.

Soorae [319] reported on a similar case involving synchronous bilateral squamous cell carcinomas. The patient showed no evidence of recurrence nine months after a two-stage bilateral lobectomy. In recent years we personally have operated on another three patients with synchronous bilateral carcinomas, owing largely to the favorable results described above. In one case the tumors were of different histologic types. All three patients survived at least two years.

The AJCC addresses this problem in the second edition of the *Manual for Staging of Cancer* [2a] and offers the following suggestions:

"Multiple synchronous tumors..., if they are of the same cell type, may be separate primaries, or one may be the primary and the other a metastasis. If there is evidence that both are primary

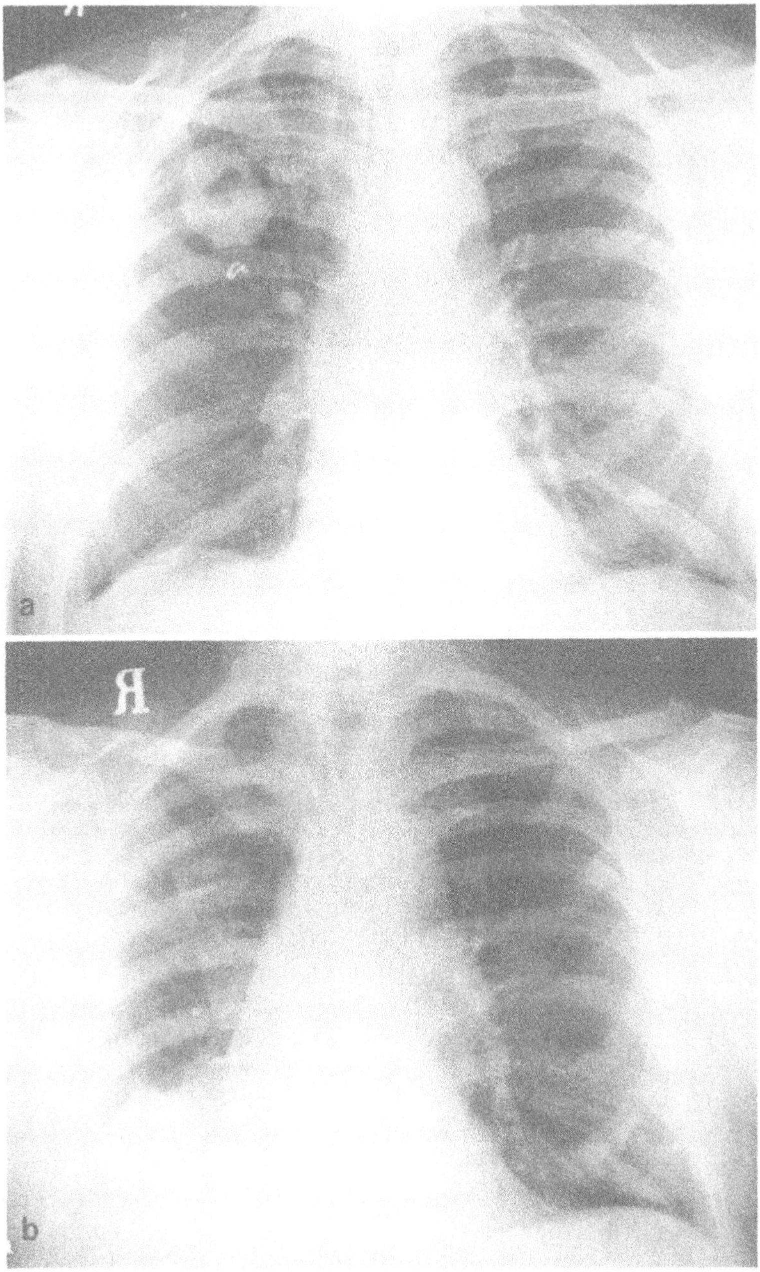

Fig. 21 a–c. Radiographic sequence showing synchronous tumors of identical histology. Patient B. W., m., 65 years of age: squamous cell carcinoma of the right upper lobe and left lower lobe (latter involvement was missed). **a** Radiograph prior to right lobectomy. **b** Conspicuous coin lesion is visible 6 weeks postoperatively

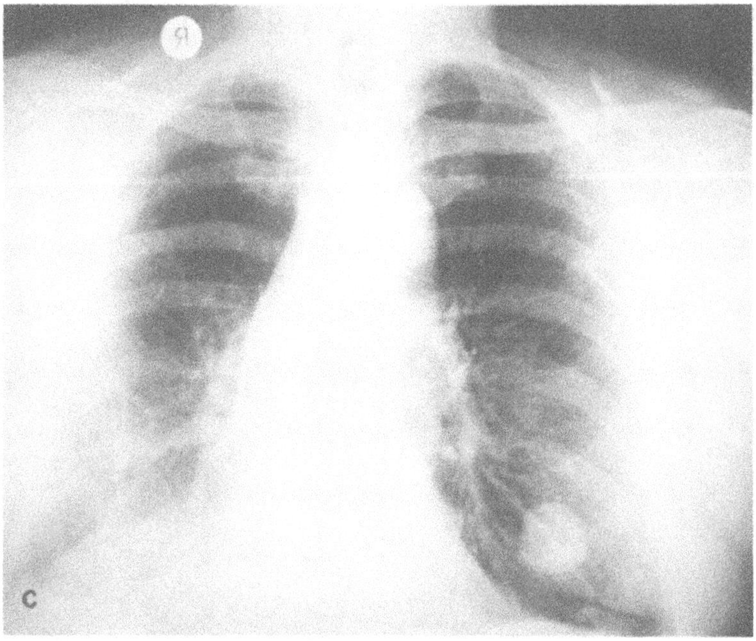

Fig. 21. c Rapid enlargement of the lesion is apparent within 6 months. Eight years after second lobectomy of the left lower lobe, patient is free of recurrence

lesions, they should be staged separately even though they are of the same cell type. If there is inadequate evidence to support a diagnosis of separate primary cancers and the "metastatic lesion" is in the contralateral lung, the designation M1 should be used. If both lesions are in the same lung, it is recommended that the designation T2 be used unless there is evidence of T3 disease. This recommendation is based on preliminary unpublished data suggesting that such cases have a relatively favorable prognosis following surgical treatment."

From our own limited experience we can support the last statement of this quote (favorable prognosis with surgery), but in actual practice (1976 and 1977) we preferred to classify these cases as $M1_{pul}$, which constitutes stage III disease. Today we still see certain difficulties in following the recommendations of the AJCC. In patients with carcinomas of the same histologic type occurring in different lobes, the option of resecting both lesions may be prohibited on functional grounds, and so it is questionable whether the designation T2 is a fair characterization. In the absence of concomitant lymph node involvement, one would have to assign such patients to stage I. Because we are dealing with a population that underwent surgery, we cannot estimate the number of patients denied surgical resection based on the finding of multiple lesions. The decision becomes extremely difficult if not two but three or more lesions are identified. Thus, we still prefer to assume that two lesions of the same cell type represent an M1 situation unless there is compelling evidence to the contrary.

Metachronous Tumors

Our experience with secondary resections of metachronous tumors is based on case data from six patients in the present series (Table 35) and from five other patients outside the series who were operated on in subsequent years. Two patients had had their primary operations 11 years and 15 years previously. In the remaining four patients, the primary and secondary operations were both performed during the period of the study. The most recent secondary operation was in 1983.

In all six patients the primary and secondary tumors were of the same cell type. In three cases the tumors were on opposite sides, and in three cases they were ipsilateral.

If we assume that highly differentiated cancers with doubling times of 100 days or longer may remain clinically and radiologically silent for more than 10 years [33], we may be justified in assuming that metachronous tumors are the expression of the same malignant disease even if a period of 15 years has elapsed between their diagnoses. On the other hand, Merrick et al. [219] point out that carcinogenic stimuli and endogenous predisposition are not affected by the primary tumor resection, and that this could account for the de novo occurrence of a second tumor. It may be some time before this question is finally resolved.

Table 35. Secondary resections for metachronous pulmonary carcinomas of identical histology

No.	Pat.	Histology	1st operation y, age, type	2nd operation y, age, type	Interval	Course following 2nd operation
1.	B.E., m	Adeno	1961/35 yrs. LUL lobectomy	1976/50 yrs. RUL lobectomy	15 yrs.	Died 25 months later from diffuse spread
2.	S.H., m	Adeno	1967/41 yrs. RML lobectomy	1978/52 yrs residual pneumonect.	11 yrs.	Surviving 7 yrs. without signs of recurrence
3.	M.R., m[a]	Adeno	1974/60 yrs. LUL lobectomy	1980/66 yrs. residual pneumonect.	5.5 yrs.	Died from contralateral recurrence after 16 months
4.	L.E., m[b]	Squam.	1975/70 yrs. LUL lobectomy	1981/76 yrs. RLL lobectomy	6.5 yrs.	Surviving 4 yrs. without signs of recurrence, well compensated respiration
5.	Z.B., m	Squam.	1976/59 yrs RUL lobectomy	1981/64 yrs. residual pneumonect.	5 yrs.	Surving 4 yrs. without signs of recurrence
6.	R.F., m	Squam	1977/62 yrs. LUL lobectomy	1983/68 yrs. RUL sleeve resection	6 yrs.	Surviving 21 months, possible signs of recurrence (mediastinal)

LUL left upper lobe, RUL right upper lobe, RLL right lower lobe, RML right middle lobe

[a] Fig. 22

[b] Fig. 23

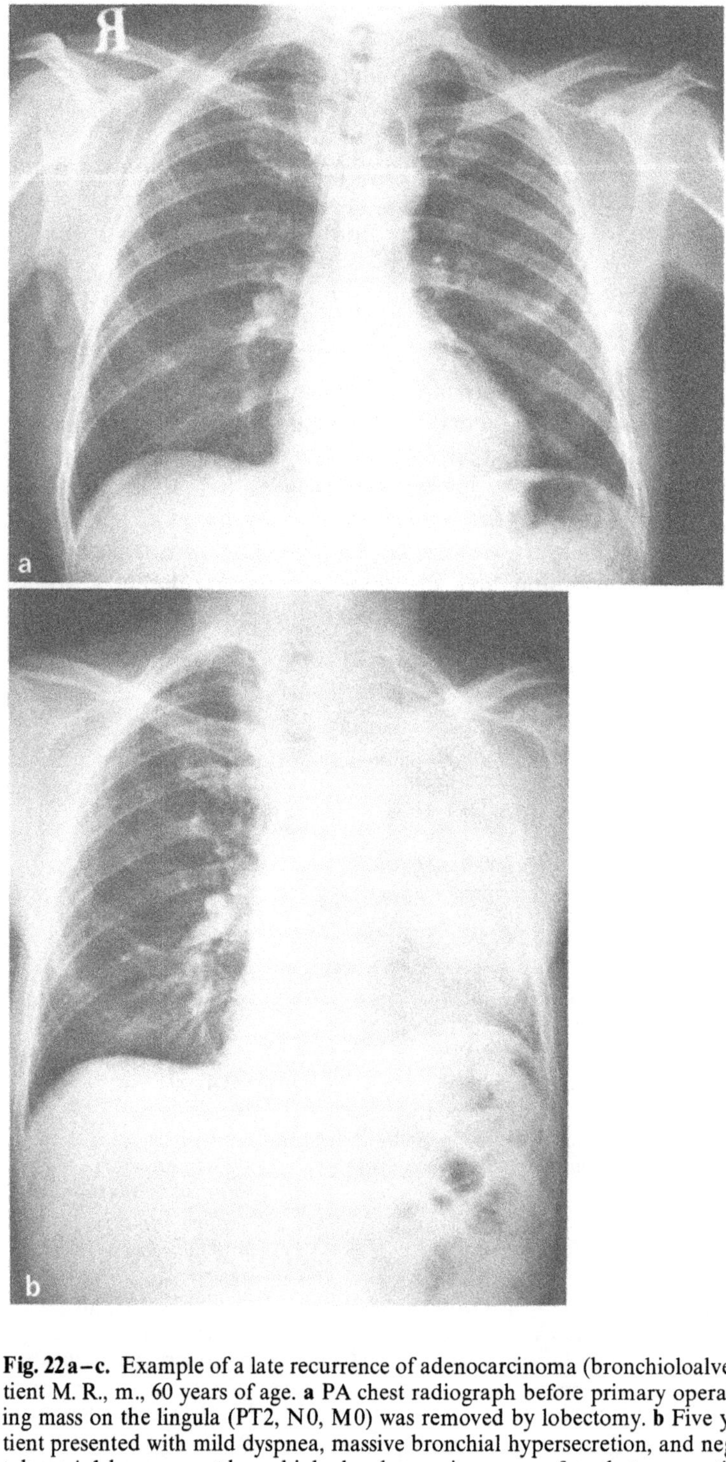

Fig. 22 a–c. Example of a late recurrence of adenocarcinoma (bronchioloalveolar variant). Patient M. R., m., 60 years of age. **a** PA chest radiograph before primary operation. The liquefying mass on the lingula (PT2, N0, M0) was removed by lobectomy. **b** Five years later the patient presented with mild dyspnea, massive bronchial hypersecretion, and negative sputum cytology. A 1-kg recurrent bronchioloalveolar carcinoma was found at reoperation

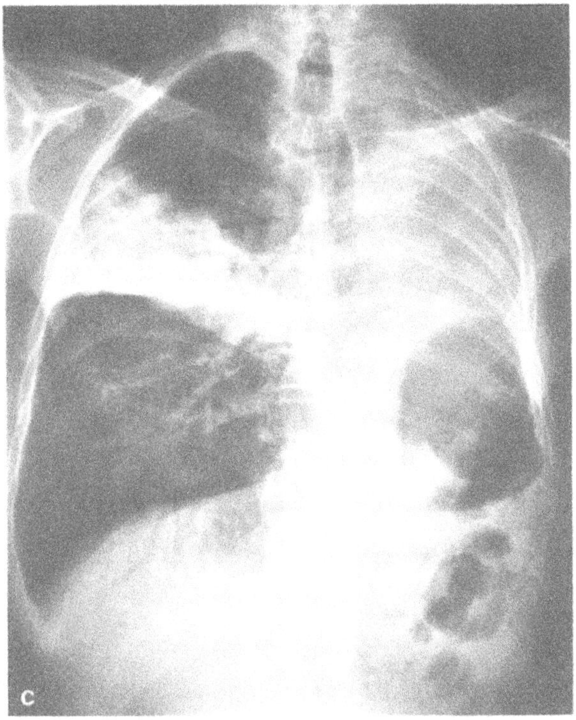

Fig. 22. c Chest radiograph 13 months after left residual pneumonectomy shows diffuse carcinosis on the right side with atelectasis or tumor infiltration of S3. The patient died 4 weeks after this film was taken, 7 years after the primary resection

Reoperation was an acceptable option in our patients because the prior resections had left them with a satisfactory level of pulmonary function. In both patients whose primary operations were done more than 10 years previously, mediastinoscopy was performed during the preoperative work-up. In the four remaining cases, mediastinoscopy had already been performed before the first operation and was not repeated.

A special problem arose in patient R. F. (No. 6 in Table 35), who had undergone a left upper lobectomy in 1977. The new carcinoma was localized in the orifice of the right upper lobar bronchus and had spread to the main bronchus, necessitating a sleeve resection. By itself, the left lower lobe provided inadequate gas exchange for carrying out the bronchial anastomosis on the right side. The solution was to ventilate the left side (lower lobe) with conventional positive pressure (IPPV) and pass a catheter through the second lumen of the Robert Shaw tube for high-frequency jet ventilation of the right lower and middle lobes [119a]. In this way the anastomosis could be performed easily and safely.

In most publications on the surgical treatment of lung cancer, no reference is made to the surgery of second tumors. An exception is the article by Overholt

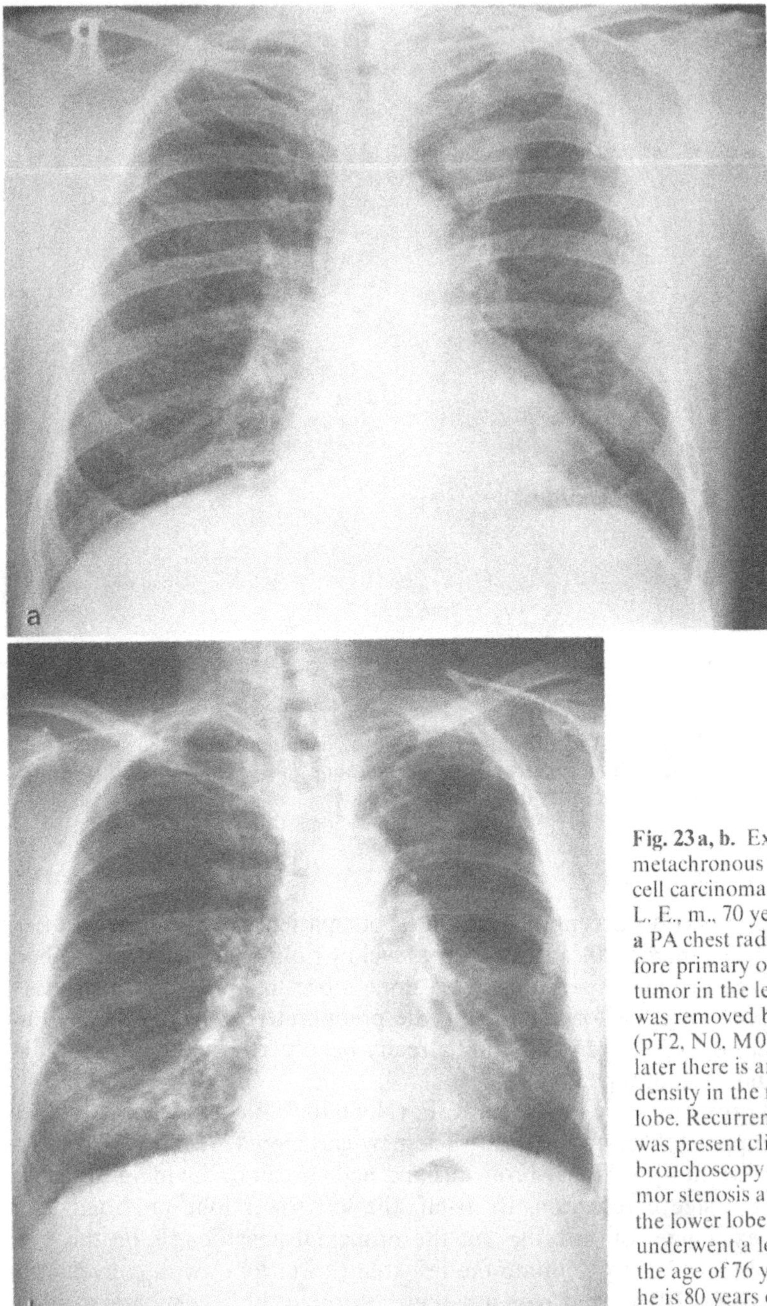

Fig. 23 a, b. Example of metachronous squamous cell carcinomas. Patient L. E., m., 70 years of age. **a** PA chest radiograph before primary operation. The tumor in the left upper lung was removed by lobectomy (pT2, N0, M0). **b** Six years later there is an infiltrative density in the right lower lobe. Recurrent pneumonia was present clinically, and bronchoscopy showed tumor stenosis at the inlet to the lower lobe. The patient underwent a lobectomy at the age of 76 years; today he is 80 years old and free of recurrence

et al. [249], who report on 96 secondary operations in a series of 1848 patients; this corresponds to an incidence of 5%. In four patients, pneumonectomies were performed after a previous contralateral segmentectomy, or segmental resections were performed after a previous pneumonectomy. The article furnishes no information on the immediate and long-term postoperative course.

Martini and Melamed [208] report on 50 cases of synchronous and metachronous tumors, 20 of which had different histologies. Thirty-four patients underwent reoperations or bilateral operations. One patient with a primary pneumonectomy died after a secondary lobectomy. A total of seven patients died within one month after resection or exploration.

Schulte et al. [292] and Schulte and Juenemann [293] report on secondary operations that were performed in 1.6% and 2.2% of surgical patients, respectively. Few if any details are given on the nature of the recurrence and secondary operations, but the figures include reinterventions for inadequate resections and operations for extrapulmonary metastases.

Gabler and Liebig [89] report survival times of several years for 3 of 17 reoperated patients. The incidence of second operations was 1.5%.

Survival Times with Multifocal Lung Tumors

In our discussion of staging (p. 24f.) we mentioned that the group of patients assigned postoperatively to stage III included 8 cases designated as $M1_{pul}$. (Note: Two of these would be classified as stage III solely on the basis of advanced lymphatic spread). It is worthwhile to investigate the prognostic significance of these multifocal or metastatic carcinomas, even with our limited case numbers, for it is anticipated that the greater routine use of computed tomography will increase the frequency with which these tumors are detected preoperatively.

First, we note that metastases in the same lobe or same lung were somewhat more common with adenocarcinomas (7.5%) than with squamous cell carcinomas (3%). Of the eight patients who had this pattern, seven underwent surgical resection, and one was technically inoperable. Of the patients who underwent lung resections, one died postoperatively from pulmonary embolism (with autopsy showing no metastatic or residual tumor); hence long-term observations are available for only six patients.

Four patients died between 27 and 31 months after surgery (average 29.5 months). One pneumonectomized patient had to be treated for intercurrent brain metastases and died six years postoperatively from his underlying disease. One patient, who also underwent pneumonectomy, has lived 7½ years without a recurrence.

Because autopsy records are available for all the patients, it is known that four succumbed to extensive pulmonary and extrapulmonary metastasis. A fifth patient died from a new pulmonary carcinoma with a different histology (first tumor was adenocarcinoma, second was squamous cell carcinoma).

Experience with Small Cell Undifferentiated Carcinomas

Results within this Series

Small cell undifferentiated carcinoma is less frequently encountered in surgical populations than other forms of lung cancer because of its rapid growth rate and its propensity for early metastasis. Fourteen of our 206 surgical patients had this carcinoma (6.8%), and it was present in 4 of the 189 patients who underwent lobectomy or pneumonectomy (2.1%). There were only five cases where surgery was undertaken with foreknowledge of the tumor histology.

The high rate of exploratory thoracotomies makes it clear that the resectability of small cell carcinoma may be questionable even before there is clinical evidence of dissemination. It should be noted, however, that when the histologic diagnosis was established by intraoperative frozen section examinations, restraint was exercised by refraining from an *extended* resection that might otherwise have been indicated.

As Table 36 shows, even patients who had exploratory thoracotomies survived up to 17 months on postoperative cytostatic therapy, which was made possible by intraoperative histologic findings. This was especially true during the second half of the reporting period.

In two patients, complete and therefore potentially curative resections were achieved. One of these patients died from a central pulmonary embolism after secondary abdominal complications (see p. 77), and the second patient developed a recurrence at 4½ years and survived almost 2 years longer on chemotherapy and radiation.

Our very limited experience with the surgical treatment of small cell undifferentiated carcinoma confirms the notoriously grim prognosis for these patients, but it also confirms the prolonged recurrence-free interval that can be obtained in isolated cases [21, 39, 205, 254, 307, 313].

On the Controversy Surrounding the Surgical Treatment of Undifferentiated Small Cell (Oat Cell) Carcinoma

The very poor success rate of the surgical (local) treatment of small cell carcinoma [84] has led many to interpret this form of lung cancer as a systemic disease process and to regard surgical resection as an obsolete measure. As early as 1969 Wulff [366] noted the attitude of "therapeutic nihilism" that existed toward the oat cell type of small cell carcinoma.

Looking at Table 37, which lists 19 references that cite 5-year results of the surgical resection of oat cell cancers, one is struck first by the small numbers of resections, and then by the great diversity in the success rates. In many reports small cell undifferentiated carcinomas are classed as one of a group of "anaplastic" cancers with markedly higher survival rates. These reports are not considered here.

Table 36. Small cell bronchial carcinomas (chronologic)

Year of op.	Preop. histol.	Mediastino-scopy	Bone marrow biopsy	Operation	Surv.	Autopsy	Remarks
1972	+	None	None	EXPLOR.	6 weeks	0	
1972	+	Neg. elsewhere	Neg.	EXPLOR.	4 months	+	Radio- and chemotherapy
1972	0	None	None	EXPLOR.	8 months	0	Radiotherapy
1973	0	Neg.	Neg.	EXPLOR.	7 months	+	Chemotherapy
1974	0	Neg.	Neg.	Lobect.	4 weeks	+	Ulcer bleeding, pulm. embolism, no metastases at autopsy
1974	0	None	Unclear	EXPLOR.	4 months	0	Radiotherapy
1974	+	Neg.	Neg.	EXPLOR.	6 months	+	Chemotherapy
1975	0	Neg. elsewhere	Neg.	Pneumonect.	25 months	+	Chemotherapy
1975	0	Neg.	None	EXPLOR.	6 months	+	Radiotherapy, no tumor at autopsy
1975	0	Neg.	Neg.	Pneumonect.	15 months	0	Chemotherapy
1977	0	Neg. elsewhere	None	EXPLOR.	11 months	+	Chemotherapy
1977	0	None	None	EXPLOR.	15 months	0	Sup. vena cava bypass, chemo- and radiotherapy
1978	+	Neg.	Neg.	Pneumonect.	76 months	0	Recurrence after 4 yrs, then chemotherapy and radiation
1978	+	Neg.	Neg.	EXPLOR.	17 months	+	Chemotherapy

Table 37. Published data on five-year survival rates after resection of small cell undifferentiated carcinoma

Author(s)	Resections	5-year survivors (n)
Ashor et al., 1975 [13]	21	0
Coman, 1974 [57]	20	5
Feinstein et al., 1974 [78]	10	3 (19%)
Greschuchna, 1978 [102]	66	(16%)
Higgins et al., 1975 [132]	11	(36%)
Kaiser, 1979 [164]	20	0
Kirsh et al., 1972 [171]	4	1 (25%)
Kirsh et al., 1976 [173]	8	3 (37%)
Mack et al., 1980 [205]	17	4 (25%)
Overholt et al., 1975 [249]	92	0
Mountain, 1977 [228]	41	0
Paulson, 1968 [253]	?	9 (6%)
Paulson and Reisch, 1976 [254]	45	0
Rubinstein et al., 1979 [280]	5	1 (20%)
Salzer, 1970 [288]	2	(9%)
Shore and Paneth, 1980 [307]	40	(27%)
Watson and Schottenfeld, 1968 [352]	27	(8%)
Wellons et al., 1968 [356]	4	1 (25%)
Wilkins et al., 1978 [363]	5 (N 0)	2 (40%)
	19 (N 1)	0

In contrast to the essentially pessimistic attitude toward the surgical treatment of this cancer, definite optimism has emerged with regard to chemotherapy used alone or in conjunction with radiation [11, 143]. The sensitivity of the tumor to cytostatic drugs and radiation has even raised hopes of effecting permanent cures – yet another reason for rejecting surgery as a treatment method.

It is known that combinations of cytostatic agents can induce remissions in 30%–90% of patients treated [99, 240]. On the other hand, the hoped-for goal of a permanent cure has not been realized. An enormous number of chemotherapeutic regimens have been devised, each involving various combinations of two to six cytostatic agents which may be given in conjunction with local radiotherapy or irradiation of the brain [43, 56, 67, 99, 296].

Chemotherapy and radiotherapy are known to cause side effects, but authors rarely give specific numerical data on associated morbidity or mortality. An exception is Brereton et al. [36], who report a 20% incidence of therapy-related deaths in a series of 50 patients. Minna et al. [222] estimate a mortality of 10% during the early remission phase even when the tumor is of limited extent and the patient's general health is good.

Recently there has been a reevaluation of the role of surgical resection in the management of small cell carcinoma. The view of Shields et al. [306] that oat cell cancers should be resected in the absence of lymph node metastases is today being adopted by many oncologists [206] either as a dominant therapy in the few cases where the cancer is detected early, or as an adjuvant to other therapies (Livingston et al. [195]: cytoreductive surgery).

Other observations seem to indicate that local recurrence and subsequent metastasis can occur despite a radiologically complete remission even while the patient is receiving systemic therapy. Autopsy studies confirm that chemotherapy and radiotherapy may be followed by the appearance of recurrent and metastatic growths that exhibit a non-small cell histology [1, 212]. This might be attributable to an alteration of tumor histology by the therapy, or perhaps to a heterogenous composition of the primary tumor, in which only the small cell component was eradicated.

Unfortunately, there is little reason to expect that more patients will be diagnosed in the early stage of their disease than is presently the case, although Shackney et al. [298] believe that, contrary to previous assumptions, the doubling time of small cell undifferentiated carcinomas is not very different from that of large cell and squamous cell carcinomas, and thus that early diagnosis could be of definite value.

Greco and Oldham [99] concede that a combination of surgical resection and chemotherapy might be the optimum treatment for small cell carcinomas of the lung. The results of Karrer et al. [166, 167], with a better than 30% 5-year survival rate, are reason for pursuing this approach further.

Recently the Lung Cancer Cooperative Group of the EORTC (European Organization for Research on Treatment of Cancer), under the direction of Goldstraw and colleagues [98 b], initiated a randomized prospective study on chemotherapy and resection versus resection alone for stage I small cell carcinoma of the lung (EORTC 08843). The EORTC is also preparing a study on adjuvant resection after induction chemotherapy in limited-disease small cell lung cancer [93 a].

Appraisal of Survival Results

In the introduction to our study we noted the difficulty of comparing published results on the surgical treatment of bronchial carcinoma. We alluded to the problem of the unambiguous characterization of a patient population, and we attempted to find a solution. It would be inconsistent for us to use the figures from the 6 publications listed in Table 38 as a measure of the quality of surgical work. For one thing, the studies were chosen arbitrarily to serve mainly as examples with which to compare the time frame and scope of our own investigation (p. 3). For another, even a cursory look at the table will show a lack of uniformity in the kinds of data that are reported. Great care must be taken, therefore, in the interpretation of apparent differences.

With regard to the frequency of exploratory thoracotomies, only the figure of 10.8% reported by Kirsh et al. [173] is comparable to our own (8.0%) – this despite the authors' statement that mediastinoscopy was *not* used to screen surgical candidates. The rate of exploratory thoracotomies is highest (though by no

Table 38

Author(s) reporting period	Patient selection	*n*	Exploratory thoracotomies	Mortality	5-year survivors	Mortality incl.
Becker et al. [20] 1960–1974 (collaborative study)	All pats. examined	4480			22.6%	?
	All pats. followed	2366				
	Lobectomies	375		15.0%		
	Pneumonectomies	550		32.0%		
	Stage I squam	121			33.0%	
	adeno	14			36.0%	
	anaplastic	29			38.0%	
Gütgemann et al. 1952–1971 [103]	All patients	855	30.2%			
(staging system not comparable)	Resections	597		24.9%	27.0%	?
Kirsh et al. [173] 1959–1969	All patients	437		6.0%		
	All operations	441	10.8%			
	Curative resect.	371				
	N0 cases				49.3%	
	Hilar LN metast.				31.1%	?
	Mediast. LN metast.				23.1%	
Megevand et al. 1967–1976 [216]	All patients	253	19.4%	9.9%		
	Stage I	100			43.2%	Yes
	Stage II	45			18.1%	Yes
	Stage III	108			4.9%	Yes
Mountain u. Hermes [229]	All resections	794	None	?		
	Stage I	330			53.0%	Yes
	Stage II	103			29.0%	Yes
	Stadium III	361			16.0%	Yes
Wilkins et al. [363] 1964–1970	All patients	322	24%			
	Resections	245		7.8%		
	Pneumonectomies	77		9.1%	26.9%	Yes
	Partial resections	168		7.5%		
	Without LN metast.	152			42.2%	Yes
	With LN metast.	85			15.0%	Yes
Own series 1972–1978	All patients	206	8%			
	All resections	187[b]		5.7%	39.5%	Yes
	Pneumonectomies	69		7.1%	39.0%	Yes
	Lobectomies	118		2.5%[a]	39.8%	Yes
	Stage I	91			53.8%	Yes
	Stage II	43			34.9%	Yes
	Stadium III	53			18.9%	Yes

[a] 30-Day mortality (hospital mortality 4%)

[b] Total number of patients minus expl. thoracotomies and 1 patient lost to follow-up

means unusual for older publications) in the series of Guetgemann et al. [103]. In the collaborative study of 16 German clinics [20] and in the study by Mountain and Hermes [229], whose time frame is not specified, no data are given on the incidence of thoracotomies performed without resection. Even a thorough perusal of the texts fails to explain why such large discrepancies exist from one study to the next.

Figures on primary mortality show a similarly large variation. They show no apparent correlation with the periods in which the studies were performed. The difference is most striking when we compare the contemporary studies of Becker et al. [20], Guetgemann et al. [103], and Kirsh et al. [173]. The mortality rate in our own series must be regarded as acceptable, but it does not represent progress over the results obtained by Kirsh et al. between 1959 and 1969, assuming that the percentage of patients with risk factors was similar.

If we examine the results in terms of the percentage of five-year survivors, we notice a striking correlation with the stage of the cancer. Only Megevand et al. [216] and Mountain and Hermes [229] use a classification that conforms to the TNM definitions of the UICC and AJCC; however, satisfactory analogies can be made from the reports of Kirsh et al. [173], Wilkins et al. [363], and, for stage I cases, Becker et al. [20]. It is not always clear whether operative mortality was included in calculations of survival rates. For patients with stage I or N0-stage disease, the reported 5-year survival rates range between 33% and 53%. Practically identical results appear in the studies of Kirsh et al. (49.3%), Mountain and Hermes (53%), and in our investigation (53.8%). These 3 studies also show good agreement in the outcomes of resections of stage II cancers (31.1%, 29.0%, 34.9%) and stage III cancers (23.1%, 16.0% 18.9%). In the work of Kirsh et al., no numerical information is given on the prevalence of the different stage groupings. Stage III cases are most prevalent in the series of Mountain and Hermes and of Megevand et al., while stage I cases clearly predominate in our series and that of Wilkins et al. It is difficult to account for these discrepancies in consecutive series. They may relate to basic differences in methods of patient selection, differences in staging, or possibly differences in the completeness of follow-up for the various stage groups.

If we were to attempt a ranking of our results relative to other publications, we could say only that from the standpoint of exploratory thoracotomies, operative mortality, and five-year survival, our results are among the most satisfying that are reported in the literature. At the same time, however, we must be mindful of the pitfalls that are inherent in such a comparison.

Chapter 8

Analysis of Deaths

We took great care to ascertain the cause of death in patients who died early or late in the postoperative course. Of the 188 patients who had resective surgery, 46 are alive today – 13 years after the start of the study and 6½ years after the closure of entry. Only one patient was lost to follow-up after two years' survival. Of the 141 patients who died after surviving up to 11 years, 83 were autopsied. This represents an autopsy rate of 59%. Half of patients who underwent exploratory thoracotomy, all of whom died, also were subjected to autopsy. Thus, a total of 92 autopsy reports were available for analysis.

As for the patients who were not autopsied, there is still a good deal of information available on the circumstances of their deaths, especially with regard to the question of tumor progression and metastasis.

Evaluation of Autopsy Findings

The autopsy records on which our analysis is based were furnished mainly by the Pathologic Institute of the University of Basel, as well as by several other institutes in Switzerland.

The records were examined in an effort to detect any correlations that might exist between the incidence of local recurrences, pattern of metastasis and histologic type, and between tumor stage and length of survival.

Autopsy Findings and Tumor Histology

Among the 141 patients who died after pulmonary resection, 93 had squamous cell carcinoma, 29 had adenocarcinoma, 15 had large cell undifferentiated or nonclassifiable carcinoma, and 4 had small cell undifferentiated carcinoma. The autopsy rates for these 4 groups range between 56% and 75% (Tables 39 and 40).

Autopsy Findings in Patients with Squamous Cell Carcinoma

In the 52 autopsies performed in this group, *local recurrences* were uncovered in 17 cases. The most common site of *metastatic spread* was the thoracic lymph nodes, which in 12 cases were involved alone and in 15 cases were involved together with abdominal or other extrathoracic nodes. Invasion of the pericardium, heart, esophagus, and aorta in the presence of local recurrence was seen in 12 cases; involvement of these structures via lymphatic spread, without local recurrence, was noted in 5 cases.

The 5 most common sites of hematogenous metastasis were, in order of frequency, the bone (11), liver (10), lung (10), and adrenals (9). Five autopsied patients had brain metastases. In two patients metastasis was to the brain only and led to death at 40 and 46 months postoperatively.

When we compare the groups of autopsied patients who did and did not have local recurrences (17 per group), we find the same overall incidence of distant metastases. However, bone metastases were almost three times more pre-

Table 39. Frequency of autopsies by tumor histology

Histology	Total series	Deaths after resection	Autopsies after resection
Squamous cell	132	93 (76%)	52 (56%)
Adenocarcinoma	40	29 (72%)	19 (65%)
Large cell and other	20	15 (75%)	9 (60%)
Small cell undiff.	14	4 (100%)	3 (75%)
	206	141 (75%)	83 (59%)

Table 40. Local recurrences and metastases[a] after resection (83 autopsies) in relation to histologic type

	Squamous cell n=52	Adeno n=19	Large cell n=9	Small cell n=3
Local recurrence (bronchus)	15	4	3	–
Lymph nodes				
Regional only	10	4	2	–
Extrathoracic	15	3	3	–
Lung	9	7	2	–
Pleura	4	3	2	–
Pericardium	7	1	2	–
Heart	3	1	2	–
Aorta	2	–	–	–
Esophagus	5	–	–	–
Liver	10	4	3	1
Kidney	5	2	1	–
Adrenal	9	3	2	1
Intestine	3	1	1	–
Bone	11	4	1	–
Brain	4	5	2	–
No recurrence	14	8	2	1

[a] Only the organs most frequently involved by metastasis or invasive tumor growth are listed

valent in patients with recurrent cancer (8 vs. 3), while brain and pulmonary metastases were more common in patients who did not develop a local recurrence.

Eighteen patients showed no evidence of local recurrence or metastasis; this represents about one-third of the autopsies for squamous cell carcinoma. It should be noted, however, that the survival time in eight cases was less than six months (including operative mortality). Eight patients who showed no residua at autopsy had other malignant disease.

Autopsy Findings in Patients with Adenocarcinoma

Autopsies were performed in 65% of patients (19 of 29) dying after resection of adenocarcinoma. Local recurrences in this group (4) were considerably less common than in patients with squamous cell cancers.

Pulmonary and pleural metastases (10) were the most common local manifestation of tumor persistence. Four instances each of hematogenous spread to the liver, bone, and brain were observed. These were followed by the adrenals (3), kidney, pancreas, and thyroid (2 each), heart, spleen, and bowel (1 each). One patient died three years postoperatively from solitary metastasis to the brain. Eight of the patients were found to have no residual or metastatic carcinoma at autopsy, although six had a different cancer – in one case a squamous cell carcinoma of the contralateral lung.

Autopsy Findings in Patients with Large Cell Carcinoma

This group was small, consisting of only 9 autopsies. Three examinations showed no evidence of local recurrence. Four patients had multiple thoracic and extrathoracic metastases. Isolated brain metastases caused death in 2 patients at 2 years and 5 years postoperatively. Two patients died from new carcinomas without developing a recurrence of the lung cancer.

Autopsy Findings in Patients with Small Cell Undifferentiated Carcinoma

All four patients with this type of cancer who underwent resection died, and three were examined by autopsy. One patient, an operative mortality, had no metastases. Another patient who survived 11 months developed hepatic and adrenal metastases. The third patient survived more than four years free of disease, dying from a clinically apparent local recurrence that was controlled for another two years with chemotherapy and radiation.

Table 41. Local recurrences and metastases after resection (83 autopsies) in relation to tumor stage (pTNM)

	Tumor stage postoperative/posthistologic		
	I (n=31)	II (n=19)	III (n=33)
Local recurrence	7	8	9
Lymph nodes			
Regional only	5	6	5
Extrathoracic	5	9	7
Lung	7	5	6
Pleura	3	3	3
Pericardium	3	3	4
Heart	0	3	3
Aorta	1	0	1
Esophagus	1	1	2
Liver	6	5	7
Kidney	1	4	3
Adrenal	2	6	6
Intestine	3	1	1
Peritoneum	2	1	1
Bone	4	6	6
Brain	5	2	4
No recurrence	12	2	11[a]

[a] Seven autopsies within 3 months after resection

Autopsy Findings and Stage of Disease

Surprisingly, Table 41 suggests that there are no differences among the three groups, in particular between stage I and stage III cases. However, one must take into account that the stage III group includes seven autopsies of early deaths (cf. p. 102). In any case, it seems remarkable to us that, in more than half of those patients classified as stage I at the time of resection (T1 or T2, N0, M0), autopsy revealed recurrent local tumor growth and/or metastases. The pattern of dissemination is extremely uniform. In this respect, as Table 40 also makes clear, the effect of the postoperative interval has not been taken into account. Therefore, we have subjected the findings to additional analysis with regard to survival time.

Autopsy Findings and Duration of Survival (Table 42)

If the autopsy findings are grouped with respect to survival time, an initial observation can be made: In 11 autopsies performed within 3 months of resection of the carcinoma, there was only a single case with persistent disease as confirmed by regional lymph node metastases. Although there were numerous stage III cases in this category, it must be stressed that, with this exception, no

Table 42. Local recurrences and metastases after resection (83 autopsies) in relation to length of survival

Postoperative survival in months	n=11 ≦3	n=11 ≦6	n=13 ≦12	n=17 ≦24	n=12 ≦36	n=6 ≦60	n=13 ≦120
Local recurrence	–	4	7	7	2	–	2
Lymph nodes							
Regional	1	1	3	1	5	2	3
Extrathoracic	–	4	4	9	3	–	1
Lung	–	2	3	4	5	2	2
Pleura	–	1	2	4	1	–	1
Pericardium	–	1	4	3	1	–	1
Heart	–	1	2	2	1	–	–
Aorta	–	1	–	1	–	–	–
Esophagus	–	2	–	2	1	–	–
Liver	–	1	6	6	4	–	1
Kidney	–	3	2	1	1	–	1
Adrenal	–	1	5	5	3	–	1
Intestine	–	0	2	1	1	–	1
Bone	–	3	2	6	2	1	2
Brain	–	1	–	5	2	1	2
No recurrence	10	5	3	3	2	2	0

other overt tumor growth was detected by routine autopsy. In other words, the clinical diagnosis and intraoperative opinion were in accordance with the post mortem findings.

The rate of local recurrences seems to be rather independent of survival time, and the same applies to lymphatic spread. However, after 1–3 years, we do observe rather a high frequency of hematogenous metastases. In particular, it is disillusioning that one-third of patients surviving from 5 to 10 years succumb from tumor progression.

Multiple Carcinomas Discovered at Autopsy

When we speak of late mortality after lung cancer surgery or of death rates, there is usually a tacit assumption that death is causally related to the malignant disease or to the cardiorespiratory stress imposed by surgery.

As the tables on the autopsy findings indicate, 29 of the 83 patients showed no residua from their lung cancer. If we subtract the 11 early deaths on the assumption that micrometastases would not be uncovered by routine autopsy, we are left with 19 patients without tumor residua in 72 autopsies (26%).

It is significant that new malignant diseases were not an uncommon finding at postmortem examination. Without autopsy, there is a natural tendency to relate indirect evidence of a metastasis to the original lung cancer. There also is a tendency to avoid invasive studies to establish the histology of the lesion in the moribund patient.

The high autopsy rate in this population gave us a more detailed picture of conditions as they actually existed. Thus, we were able to determine that 27 additional carcinomas were present in 21 patients autopsied, and that some of these cancers either were the cause of death or were a significant contributing factor. The 21 cases are reviewed in Table 43.

It should be noted that in some cases the histologic form of the lung carcinoma was related to that of the tumor found at autopsy. However, all the tumors presented locally as primary tumors rather than metastases, and their histologies were not absolutely identical. Even so, we cannot rule out the possibility that a few of the pulmonary resections were performed for lesions that were metastatic to the lung from an extrapulmonary source. This uncertainty exists to some degree in all operative series.

Analysis of Unautopsied Cases

Autopsies were not performed in nine cancer patients who had undergone exploratory thoracotomy, and who were judged clinically to have died from progression of their underlying disease.

Of the 141 patients who died after *resection,* 58 were not autopsied. Fairly detailed information is available on 44 of these patients, because they died in hospitals.

In the six patients who died at home, cardiac death was declared in five cases, and death in a man almost 80 years old was referred to senile debility. None of these patients dying suddenly showed any signs of tumor recurrence in their follow-up examinations, which were done at most six months previously, and none exhibited unusual symptoms before their deaths. It may be assumed, then, that these patients did not die as a direct result of their malignant disease. Three patients with an advanced tumor stage at the time of resection died abroad. A causal relationship with the lung cancer is probable but not definite. In five patients we were unable to obtain information other than the time of death.

The following analysis, then, is limited to the 53 cases in which documented information was available on the circumstances of death. In the patients who died in hospital, it often was possible to get objective proof of local or metastatic tumor progression by sputum examination, bronchoscopy, pleural biopsy, and the aspiration of pleural or ascitic fluid. The cases of bony and pulmonary metastasis that were accessible to radiologic documentation also are regarded as confirmed. Table 44 shows the frequencies of the various manifestations.

Summary of the Incidence of Recurrences and Metastases in 135 Deaths

If we summarize the results of the 83 autopsies and the findings in 52 of the 58 patients not autopsied, we find that one-third of the patients who died had local recurrences of their cancers, with or without distant metastases. The most com-

Table 43. Additional malignant tumors confirmed by autopsy

Pat., age, sex, length of survival	Operated lung cancer	Second carcinoma	Third carcinoma	Fourth carcinoma	Cause of death
1. A. M., 66, w. 5 months	Adeno No recurrence	Gastric cancer diffuse metast.	–	–	2nd Carcinoma
2. H. M., 42, m. 5 months	Adeno No recurrence	Malignant small bowel polyps, diffuse metast.	–	–	2nd Carcinoma
3. P. C., 73, m. 43 months	Squamous cell No recurrence	Chron. myel. leukemia	–	–	Leukemia
4. R. H., 68, m. 16 months	Large cell No recurrence	Anaplast. thyroid cancer + metast.	–	–	2nd Carcinoma
5. R. M., 56, m. 9 months	Large cell No recurrence	Sarcoma of chest wall, bony metast.	–	–	Sarcoma
6. M. H., 60, m. 31 months	Adeno No recurrence	Papill. adenocarcinoma of pancreas, diffuse metast.	–	–	2nd Carcinoma
7. S. L., 51, m. 31 months	Adeno No recurrence	Squamous cell cancer of lung, regional metast.	–	–	2nd Carcinoma
8. B. H., 62, m. 12 months	Squamous cell No recurrence	Adenocarcinoma of prostate no metast.	–	–	Coronary heart disease
9. H. A., 65, m. 4 months	Adeno No recurrence	Adenocarcinoma of prostate, no metast.	–	–	Pneumonia after laparotomies
10. Z. J., 52, m. 21 months	Squamous cell	Squamous cell cancer of lung	–	–	2nd Carcinoma, alcoholic hepatopathy
11. K. A., 56, m. 6 months	Squamous cell Local recurrence + metastasis	Adenocarcinoma of colon, hepatic metast.	Circumferential rectal papilloma	–	2nd Carcinoma
12. S. P., 68, m. 6 months	Squamous cell Local recurrence	Stenosing carcinoid of small bowel	–	–	2nd Carcinoma
13. T. M., 54, m. 24 months	Alveolar cell Diffuse metast.	Papill. thyroid cancer, no metast.	(Cavernous hemangiomas of liver and spine)	–	Meningeosis carcinomatosa (lung carcinoma)

14. T.P., 63, m. 5 months	Squamous cell No recurrence	Urothelial bladder cancer	Adenocarcinoma of lung	–	Bladder carcinoma
15. B.R., 66, m. 0	Squamous cell No recurrence	Microscop. squamous cell cancer of contralateral lung	Adenocarcinoma of lung	–	Operative mortality
16. S.W., 66, m. 34 months	Large cell No recurrence	Adenocarcinom of pancreas	Multicentric prostatic cancer	–	Pneumonia after periph. pulmonary embolisms
17. S.G., 63, m. 35 months	Squamous cell Metastasis to 1 lymph node	Sigmoid cancer	Hypernephroid renal cancer	–	Sigmoid anastomotic leak
18. G.E., 63, m. 13 months	Adeno No recurrence	Reticulosarcoma of brain, metast. to liver and spleen	Squamous cell cancer of lower lip, op.	Basal cell cancer of cheek, op.	Sarcoma
19. W.H., 62, m. 69 months	Squamous cell	Melanoma (foot)	–	–	Diffuse metastasis from melanoma
20. S.E., 63, m. 10.5 yrs.	Squamous cell	Squamous cell cancer (tongue)	–	–	2nd Carcinoma, metastases
21. B.H., 68, m.	Squamous cell	Vocal cord cancer	Large cell cancer of oppos. lung	–	3rd Carcinoma, diffuse metastasis

Table 44. Clinical findings at time of death in 52 patients who underwent lung cancer surgery

Local recurrence	18
Lymph node metastases	9
Pulmonary metastases	9
Liver metastases	5
Bony metastases	9
Brain metastases	4
Other malignant diseases	4
No signs of recurrence	14

mon sites of hematogenous spread were the lung and bone. Metastases to the liver and brain also were a common finding in the autopsied patients, but they were diagnosed less frequently during clinical evaluation.

The three times greater incidence of second and third carcinomas in the autopsied patients is based on the discovery of clinically irrelevant carcinomas (e.g., prostatic cancer without metastases) and the finding of tumors which, at autopsy, proved to be independent of the primary lung tumor.

Both series contain similar percentages of patients who died without demonstrable recurrence of their tumor. This was the case in 42 of the 135 cases evaluated, or approximately 32%.

From a therapeutic standpoint, it is important to note that of the 92 patients who died with recurrent or metastatic disease, 7 had metastasis confined to the brain. Thus, approximately one-third of all brain metastases were solitary, regardless of the histology of the primary tumor (cf. [225, 334]).

Finally we sought to determine how many of the patients who did not die from tumor progression died as an *indirect* result of their disease. This may be postulated for the eight patients in our series who were classified as operative deaths. Two pneumonias after pneumonectomy and two postpneumonectomy cases of clinically diagnosed right heart failure also may be viewed as causally linked to the carcinoma treatment. Further details are given in Table 45.

Our investigations on the postoperative behavior of the malignant disease as established from autopsy findings indicate the following:

1. Findings in the early postoperative autopsies were consistent with the tumor stage that had been identified preoperatively and intraoperatively. Regional lymph node metastases were found in only 1 of 11 patients who died and were autopsied within 3 months.

2. Nearly one-third of the patients died with no clinical or autopsy residua of their primary lung cancer. This was true in almost 50% of the patients who had been operated in stage I.

The first observation conflicts with the findings of other authors [23, 210, 213, 324, 346, 352]. Matthews et al. [210, 213] reviewed 202 autopsies from several operative series that had been performed within 4 weeks after a presumably curative resection. In 35% of cases they found a persistence of malignant disease (Table 46). Bell [23] found 7 cases of occult metastasis in 22 autopsies performed within 4 weeks of surgery. Vincent et al. [346] reported unexpected metastases and local, residual tumor in 11 of 33 early postoperative deaths. In a study by Spjut and Mateo [324], a similarly high incidence of residual tumor and distant metastases (73%) was noted in 87 autopsies, 15 of which were performed in the first postoperative month. Weiss and Gillick [353] report finding metastases in 11 of 35 autopsies performed within 1 month of resection.

Almost all of the studies cited above are distinguished by relatively large numbers of autopsies, and only the 1965 study of Spjut and Mateo is comparable in scope to our own. The problem with these studies is that none are based on consecutive operative series, but rather on the evaluation of autopsy cases drawn from various clinics. Thus, they are unable to give information on

Table 45. Causes of death in 42 patients free of recurrence

Operative mortality	8
Second malignant disease	18
Nasal + 2nd lung cancer (81)[a]	
2nd lung cancer (31, 60, and 88)	
Leukemia (43)	
Pancreatic cancer (31)	
Lingual cancer (21, 29, and 126)	
Thyroid cancer (16)	
Sarcomas (9 and 13) of brain/soft tissues	
Bladder cancer (5)	
Cancer of stomach (5) and small bowel (5)	
Prostatic cancer (4 and 12)	
Melanoma (69)	
Suicide	1
Cerebrovascular accidents (1.5, 6, 50, and 74)	4
Bilateral pneumonia (45)	1
Pneumonia after pneumonectomy (3 and 80)	2
Rupture of abdominal aortic aneurysm (22)	1
Pulmonary embolism in glomerulonephritis (1.5)	1
Myocardial infarction after lobectomy (3, 9, and 19)	3
Cardiac failure after pneumonectomy (40 and 86)	2
Senile debility (87)	1

[a] Numbers in parentheses indicate survival in months

Table 46. Incidence of residual tumor after curative resection in 202 patients who died and were autopsied within 30 days[a]

Histology	Number of patients	Tumor persistence	Local only	Distant metastases
Squamous cell	131	44 (33%)	22	22
Adeno	30	13 (43%)	1	12 (40%)
Large cell	22	3 (14%)	–	3 (14%)
Small cell	19	13 (70%)	1	12 (63%)
Total	202	73 (35%)	24	49

[a] After Metthews et al.: *Cancer Chemotherapy Reports 4*, 63, 1973

preoperative diagnosis or on the principles that were followed in carrying out the resections. The finding of residual tumor after an ostensibly curative resection should be exceptional if proper care is taken to confirm the adequacy of the resection by histologic means. With careful mediastinoscopic exploration and intraoperative frozen section examinations of random lymph node specimens, it should also be possible to limit greatly the incidence of residual lymphatic metastases. Indeed, it must be asked whether the elective surgery of lung carcinoma is at all justified without the availability of intraoperative frozen section examinations [9].

Our second observation, that a significant percentage of late deaths are not based on a progression of the primary malignant disease but on new malignancies, agrees with the results of Ashor et al. [13], who found that 20% of patients who survived resective surgery longer than 5 years developed a second carcinoma. R. A. Smith [313] observed that a quarter of his patients who survived longer than 10 years died from a new lung carcinoma, and he reported a total of 60 new cancers developing in long-term survivors of 1250 resections.

Finally, we attach importance to the high incidence of brain metastases found at autopsy in patients with adenocarcinoma of the lung. Of 11 patients who died from recurrent adenocarcinoma, 5 had cerebral metastases (only 4 of 30 patients with recurrent squamous cell carcinoma had these metastases). Despite the small numbers, we feel that these observations confirm the findings of Line and Deeley [194], who, in a series of 680 autopsies, noted an almost equally high incidence of brain metastases from adenocarcinoma as from small cell carcinoma (39% vs. 42%). Their study contained no information on clinical findings or therapy. Cox and Yesner [58] found brain metastases in 54% of adenocarcinoma cases. In their series, which included 400 autopsies performed after radiation therapy, the incidence of brain metastasis from adenocarcinoma even exceeded that from small cell carcinomas (45%).

As we showed in our discussion of long-term results, tumor histology in this series had no statistically apparent effect on long-term therapeutic outcomes. Accordingly, patients with adenocarcinomas had similar chances for survival or cure as patients with other lung cancers, despite the propensity of adenocarcinoma for cerebral metastasis. We believe, therefore, that the autopsy findings do not warrant expanding the preoperative diagnostic work-up to include additional brain studies, particularly since almost all brain metastases were detected only when autopsy was performed after more than 1 year of postoperative survival (cf. Table 42).

Concluding Remarks

One must be cautious when comparing our experience in a relatively small, closely followed population with results in other publications. We have described the reason for this at great length: lack of uniformity of definitions. Certainly the TNM classification is the most fully developed cancer staging system in existence today, but it, too, is in a process of continual revision and refinement. We have pointed out several areas that are in need of clarification, and in several instances we took the liberty of making our own interpretations where existing definitions seemed to be ambiguous.

Certainly it would be desirable to develop conventions that would enable aspects of surgical technique to be described in concise, uniform terms. Our suggestions on this point are by no means new and are based on terminology that has been known for many years.

In any event, the effects of surgical treatment on life expectancy are both promising and encouraging. It is difficult to speak of cures, however, because even patients who have survived for years often die as a result of their malignant disease.

In evaluating survival results, it is necessary to consider both the number of exploratory thoracotomies performed without resection and the level of surgery-related mortality. Although known risk factors such as advanced age and impaired cardiopulmonary function must be accepted to some degree when selecting patients for operation, it is possible to keep the primary mortality within limits that allow for an acceptable overall risk. The preoperative recognition of risk factors may require considerable extra effort, but in our view it is fully justified. We would not advocate a general simplification of the evaluation protocol described earlier in the text, but we have learned how to extend the boundaries of functional operability and thus recognize the potential for resectability in a greater number of surgical candidates.

With regard to oncologic screening, it is acknowledged that considerable discrepancies may exist between the clinical or preoperative tumor stage (cTNM) and the postoperative stage (pTNM). Through preoperative mediastinoscopy, at least, it has been possible to greatly decrease the incidence of "nonproductive" exploratory thoracotomies. Today our procedure for the evaluation of lung cancer patients differs from that described previously in that we dispense with mediastinoscopy if CT scans are normal, unless there is suspicion of small cell undifferentiated carcinoma. In the near future we will be able to determine whether this modification of our protocol has any deleterious effects.

As evidence for the efficacy of our diagnostic program, we note that only 1 in 10 patients who died within 3 months of operation had manifestations of carcinoma at autopsy. Admittedly the case numbers are small, but we consider this result to be more than coincidental. It remains to be seen whether the accuracy of preoperative staging can be further improved by the use of computed tomography. Experience to date indicates that this radiologic technique furnishes accurate information on tumor extent in continuity with extrapulmonary organs. It is less useful, apparently, for confirming metastatic involvement of enlarged regional lymph nodes or excluding mestatasis in nodes of normal size.

As long as alternative treatment modalities, most notably the development of more effective chemotherapeutic drugs, cannot provide a better balance between the prolongation of survival and the quality of life, surgical resection will continue to be a useful treatment even for certain advanced cancers. A review of the stage III lung cancers in our series shows that the percentage of patients surviving 5 years, at 20%, is still markedly higher than the incidence of primary mortality. It has been our experience, moreover, that the trauma of surgery is a self-limiting disturbance and that even the losses of physical stress tolerance caused by pneumonectomy are tolerated by patients with minor difficulty. On the whole, then, our results support a more aggressive approach to the management of these cancers. We also tend to consider surgery more frequently for localized recurrences and for secondary tumors of the lung, particularly since it cannot be determined whether the latter represent hematogenous metastases or autonomous carcinomas. In the cases where we elected to perform a secondary resection, our actions did not strictly conform to accepted selection criteria for curative or palliative operations. In retrospect, longevity overall was substantially prolonged by these resections, and the operative risk was not excessive.

References

1. Abeloff, M.D., Eggleston, J.C., Mendelsohn, G., Ettinger, D.S., Baylin, S.B.: Changes in morphologic and biochemical characteristics of small cell carcinoma of the lung. Am. J. Med. *66,* 757 (1979)
2. Acosta, J.L., Manfredi, F.: Selective mediastinoscopy. Chest *71,* 150 (1977)

2a. American Joint Committee (AJCC): Manual for Staging of Cancer. J. J. Lippincott, Philadelphia 1983

3. Akovbiantz, A., Äberhard, P.: Mediastinoskopie in der Diagnostik und Operabilitätsbeurteilung bei Lungenerkrankungen. Thoraxchir. *12,* 193 (1964/1965)
4. Akovbiantz, A.: Die Mediastinoskopie (Aktuelle Probleme in Chirurgie und Orthopädie 3). Huber, Bern/Stuttgart/Wien 1977
5. Alazraki, N.P., Ramsdell, J.W., Taylor, A., Friedman, P.J., Peters, R.M., Tisi, G.M.: Reliability of gallium scan chest radiography compared to mediastinoscopy for evaluating mediastinal spread in lung cancer. Am. Rev. Respir. Dis. *117,* 415 (1978)
6. Alth, G.: Die Strahlentherapie beim Bronchuskarzinom. In Denck, H., Sighart, H.: Das Bronchuskarzinom heute. Adolf Holzhausen Nfg., Wien 1980
7. American Thoracic Society, Medical Section of the National Tuberculosis and Respiratory Disease Association: Diagnostic Mediastinoscopy. Am. Rev. Respirator. Dis. *105,* 487 (1972)
8. Amgwerd, R., Largiader, F.: Zur Technik und Indikation der Mediastinoskopie bei Erkrankungen der Lungen und des Mediastinums. Helv. Chir. Acta *30,* 33 (1963)
9. Ammendick, U., Konrad, R.M.: Therapie solider Tumoren, gezeigt am Beispiel des Bronchialkarzinoms. Münch. med. Wschr. *119,* 238 (1977)
10. Arndt, R.D., Frank, C.G., Schmitz, A.L., Haveson, S.B.: Cardiac herniation with volvulus after pneumonectomy. Am. J. Roentgenol. *130,* 155 (1978)
11. Arnold, H.: Die zytostatische Behandlung des Bronchialkarzinoms. Therapiewoche *29,* 7240 (1979)
12. Ashbaugh, D.G.: Mediastinoscopy. Arch. Surg. *100,* 568 (1970)
13. Ashor, G.L., Kern, W.H., Meyer, B.W., Lindesmith, G.G., Stiles, Q.R., Turker, B.L., Jones, J.C.: Long-term survival in bronchogenic carcinoma. J. Thorac. Cardiovasc. Surg. *70,* 581 (1975)
14. Baker, R.R., Stitik, F.P., Marsh, B.R.: The clinical assessment of selected patients with bronchogenic carcinoma. Ann. Thorac. Surg. *20,* 520 (1975)
15. Baldamus, U., Ceh, M.: Verlaufsbeobachtung und Behandlungsergebnisse von 1000 Patienten mit Bronchialcarcinom. Pneumologie *145,* 164 (1970)
16. Barker, W.L., Langston, H.T., Naffah, P.: Postresection thoracic spaces. Ann. Thorac. Surg. *2,* 299 (1966)
17. Barth, H.: Die klinische Studie – Voraussetzungen für die Bewertung therapeutischer Konzepte. In Hamelmann, H., Troidl, H.: Behandlung des Bronchialkarzinoms. Georg Thieme, Stuttgart/New York 1981.
18. Beatti, E.J.: Operative mortality and five-year survival rates in men with bronchogenic carcinoma. Chest *66,* 469 (1974)
19. Becker, H., Wacha, H., Ungeheuer, E.: Pancoast-Tumor. Fortschr. Med. *95,* 2045 (1977)
20. Becker, H., Borst, H.G., Brieler, H.S., et al.: Ergebnisse der operativen Behandlung des Bronchialkarzinoms. Dtsch. Med. Wschr. *101,* 1553 (1976)
21. Belcher, J.R., Anderson, R.: Surgical treatment of carcinoma of the bronchus. Brit. Med. J. *1,* 948 (1965)

22. Belcher, J.R., Sturridge, M.F.: Thoracic surgical management. 4th ed. Baillière Tindall, London (1972)
23. Bell, J.W.: Survival and cancer of the lung. Surg. Gyn. Obstet. *118,* 839 (1964)
24. Benfield, J.R., Juillard, G.J.F., Pilch, Y.H., Rigler, L.G., Selecky, P.: Current and future concepts in lung cancer, UCLA Conference. Ann. Int. Med. *83,* 93 (1975)
25. Berardi, R.S., Malette, W.G., Dillon, M.L.: An evaluation of routine diagnostic procedures in cancer of the lung. J. Thorac. Cardiovasc. Surg. *44,* 82 (1972)
26. Berend, N., Woolcock, A.J., Marlin, G.E.: Effects of lobectomy on lung function. Thorax *35,* 145 (1980)
27. Bergh, N.P., Schersten, T.: Bronchogenic carcinoma. A follow-up study of a surgically treated series with special reference to the prognostic significance of lymph node metastases. Acta Chir. Scand. Suppl. *347* (1965)
28. Berndt, E.: Absterbekurven nach Operation wegen eines Bronchialkarzinoms. Zschr. Erkr. Atmungsorg. *132,* 253 (1970)
29. Berthoumieu, F., Henry, E., Glovaez, D., Desrez, X., Pradere, B., Fournial, G., Gaillard, J.: Troubles du rythme cardiaque après pneumonectomie. Essai de prévention. Le poumon et le coeur *34,* 49 (1978)
30. Bogusch, L.K., Travin, A.A., Semenenkow, J.L.: Transperikardiale Operationen an den Hauptbronchien und Lungengefäßen. Hippokrates, Stuttgart 1971
31. Borm, D., Backhaus, J.: Der Lungenrundherd. Ein Beitrag zur Frühdiagnostik des Bronchialkarzinoms. Med. Welt *29,* 298 (1978)
32. Borrie, J.: Management of emergencies in thoracic surgery. 2nd. ed. Appleton-Century-Crofts, New York 1972
33. Boucot, K.R., Cooper, D.A., Weiss, W.: The role of surgery in the cure of lung cancer. Arch. Intern. Med. *120,* 168 (1967)
34. Boushy, S.F., Billig, D.M., North, L.B., Helgason, A.H.: Clinical course related to preoperative and postoperative pulmonary function in patients with bronchogenic carcinoma. Chest *59,* 383 (1971)
35. Brantigan, J.W., Brantigan, C.O., Brantigan, O.C.: Biopsy of nonpalpable scalene lymph nodes in carcinoma of the lung. Am. Rev. Respir. Dis. *107,* 962 (1973)
36. Brereton, H.D., Kent, C.H., Johnson, R.E.: Chemotherapy and radiation therapy for small cell carcinoma of the lung: a remedy for post therapeutic failure. In: Muggia, F., Rozenczweig, M.: Lung cancer: progress in therapeutic research. Raven Press, New York 1979
37. Brock, R.C.: Bronchial carcinoma. Brit. Med. J. *2,* 237 (1948)
38. Brock, R.C.: Radical pneumonectomy. Thorax *15,* 7 (1960)
39. Brock, R.C.: Survival after operation for lung cancer. Brit. J. Surg. *62,* 1 (1975)
40. Brock, R.C., Whytehead, L.L.: Radical pneumonectomy for bronchial carcinoma. Brit. J. Surg. *43,* 8 (1955)
41. Brofman, B.L., Charms, B.L., Kohn, P.M., Elder, J., Newman, R., Rizika, M.: Unilateral pulmonary artery occlusion. Control studies. J. Thorac. Cardiovasc. Surg. *34,* 206 (1957)
42. Brooks, J.W.: Complications following pulmonary lobectomy. In: Cordell, R.A., Ellison, R.G., eds.: Complications of intrathoracic surgery. Little Brown & Company, Boston 1979
42a. Broughton, D.L., Gibson, C.J., Crake, T., Pearce, S.J., Leonard, R.C.F.: Gallium scanning by conventional imaging and emission computed tomography in the pretreatment evaluation of lung cancer. Thorax *40,* 96 (1985)
43. Brunner, A., Brunner, W.: Das Bronchialalveolarzellkarzinom als solitärer Rundherd. Schweiz. Med. Wschr. *107,* 211 (1977)
44. Bünemann, H., Heilmann, H.P.: Kurative Zielsetzung bei Strahlentherapie des Bronchuskarzinoms. Dtsch. Ärzteblatt *77,* 261 (1980)
45. Byrd, R.B., Carr, D.T., Miller, W.E., Payne, W.S., Woolner, L.B.: Radiographic abnormalities in carcinoma of the lung as related to histological cell type. Thorax *24,* 573 (1969)
46. Cahen, W.G.: Radical lobectomy. J. Thorac. Cardiovasc. Surg. *39,* 555 (1960)
47. Carr, D.T.: Does Staging help? In: Perspectives in Lung Cancer. F.E. Jones Memorial Symposia in Thoracic Surgery. Karger, Basel 1977
48. Carr, D.T., Mountain, C.F.: Staging Lung Cancer. In Straus M.J.: Lung Cancer; Clinical diagnosis and treatment. Grune & Stratton, New York/San Francisco/London 1977

48a. Carr, D.T., Mountain, C.F.: Staging lung cancer. In: Strauss, M.J.: Lung Cancer. Clinical diagnosis and treatment. 2nd ed. Grune & Stratton, New York 1983

48b. Carney, D.N., Matthews, M.J., Ihde, D.C.: Influence of histologic subtype of small cell carcinoma of the lung on clinical presentation, response to therapy and survival. J. Natl. Cancer Inst. *65,* 1225 (1980)

49. Castrup, W.: Die Röntgensymptomatik des Bronchialkarzinoms. Therapeut. Umschau *35,* 1010 (1978)

50. Cernik, H.: Was erreicht die operative Bronchialkarzinombehandlung heute? Zbl. Chir. *209,* 383 (1972)

51. Chamberlain, J.M., McNeill, T.M., Parnassa, P., Edsall, J.R.: Bronchogenic carcinoma: an aggressive surgical attitude. J. Thoracic Surgery *38,* 727 (1959)

52. Churg, A., Johnston, W.H., Stulbarg, M.: Small cell squamous and mixed small cell squamous-small cell anaplastic carcinomas of the lung. Am. J. Surg. Pathol. *4,* 255 (1980)

53. Clagett, O.T.: Mediastinoscopy – good or evil? J. Thorac. Cardiovasc. Surg. *60,* 754 (1970)

53a. Choi, N.C.: The role of postoperative radiation therapy in lung cancer with either metastases to regional lymph nodes (N1 or unforeseen N2) or direct invasion beyond visceral pleura (T3). In: Choi, N.C., Grillo, H.C., eds., Thoracic Oncology, Raven Press, New York 1983

54. Clarke, D.B.: Pulmonary embolism after lung surgery. In: Smith, R.E., Williams, W.G.: Surgery of the lung. The Coventry conference. Butterworths, London 1974

55. Cliffton, E.E.: Evaluation for treatment, B. criteria for operability and resectability. In Watson, W.L., ed.: Lung Cancer. A study of 5000 Memorial Hospital Cases. C.V. Mosby Company, St. Louis 1968

56. Cohen, M.H.: Bronchogenic Carcinoma. In Staquet, M.J. ed.: Randomized Trials in Cancer: a critical review in sites. Raven Press, New York 1978

57. Coman, C.: Conception actuelle du traitement chirurgical du cancer broncho-pulmonaire. Le poumon et le coeur *30,* 141 (1974)

58. Cox, J.D., Yesner, R.A.: Adenocarcinoma of the lung. Recent results from the Veterans Administration Lung Group. Am. Rev. Respirator. Dis. *120,* 1025 (1979)

59. Cutler, S.J., Ederer, F.: Maximum utilization of the life table method in analyzing survival. J. Chron. Dis. *8,* 699 (1958)

60. Daum, S., Herzog, H., Georg, R., Spillmann, B., Burckhardt, D.: Beurteilung der Lungenoperabilität vom Standpunkt der Hämodynamik im kleinen Kreislauf. Pneumonologie *144,* 266 (1971)

61. Delarue, N.C., Strasberg, S.V.: The rationale of intensive preoperative investigation in bronchogenic carcinoma. J. Thorac. Cardiovasc. Surg. *51,* 392 (1966)

62. Denck, H., Zwintz, E.: Die Operationsindikation bei Verdacht auf Bronchuskarzinom. Das „Risiko“ der Fehlbeurteilung. Pneumologie *146,* 148 (1971)

63. Denck, H., Olbert, F., Zwintz, E.: Indikationen zur Mediastinoskopie und deren Aussagewert. Langenbecks Arch. *327,* 202 (1970)

64. Deutsche Gesellschaft für Chirurgie: Praxis der Krebsbehandlung in der Chirurgie. Der Lungenkrebs. Empfehlung K 6. Thoraxchir. *26,* 381 (1978)

65. Dolton, E.G.: Combined surgery and chemotherapy for carcinoma of bronchus. Lancet *1,* 40 (1970)

66. Dunn, D., Hertel, B., Norwood, W., Nicoloff, D.M.: Bronchioloalveolar cell carcinoma of the lung: a clinicopathological study. Ann. Thorac. Surg. *26,* 241 (1978)

67. Eagan, R.T., Maurer, L.H., Forcier, J.J., Tulloh, M.: Small cell carcinoma of the lung: staging, paraneoplastic syndroms, treatment and survival. Cancer *33,* 527 (1974)

68. Ellison, L.T.: Preoperative assessment of the patient with lung cancer. In: Murray, G.F., ed.: Cancer of the lung. Stratton, New York/London 1974

69. Elmendorff v., H.: Zur Berechnung der Behandlungserfolge von Bronchuskarzinomen. Langenbecks Arch. *325,* 525 (1969)

70. Endrei, E.: Thorax Röntgen Diagnostik. II Das Lungenkarzinom. Ciba-Geigy, Basel 1979

71. Enstrom, J.E., Austin, D.F.: Interpreting cancer survival rates. Science *195,* 847 (1977)

72. Ermisch, K.: Fünfjahresergebnisse bei operativer Behandlung des Bronchialkarzinoms unter Berücksichtigung der Methode der Erstfeststellung. Zschr. Erkrank. Atmungs. Org. *133,* 170 (1970)
73. Erozan, Y.S., Frost, J.K.: Cytopathologic diagnosis of lung cancer. In: Straus, M.J., ed.: Lung Cancer. Grune & Stratton, New York 1977
74. Eule, H.: Klinische Diagnose des Bronchialkarzinoms. Ther. Umschau *35,* 999 (1978)
75. Famos, M., Hasse, J., Grädel, E.: Der Restpneumothorax nach Lungenteilresektion. Helv. Chir. Acta *47,* 33 (1980)
76. Favez, G.: Le diagnostic précose du cancer bronchique: son utilité. Schweiz. Med. Wschr. *106,* 922 (1976)
77. Feinstein, A.R., Gelfman, N.A., Yesner, R.: Observer variability in the histopathologic diagnosis of lung cancer. Am. Rev. Respir. Dis. *101,* 671 (1970)
78. Feinstein, A.R., Gelfman, N.A., Yesner, R.: The diverse effects of histopathology on manifestations and outcome of lung cancer. Chest *66,* 225 (1974)
79. Fischer, J.: Lungenfunktionsdiagnostik beim Bronchuskarzinom. Therapiewoche *29,* 7180 (1979)
80. Fischnaller, M.: Zytodiagnostik in der Pulmonologie. In: Denck, H., Sighart, H.: Das Bronchuskarzinom heute. Adolf Holzhausen Nfg., Wien 1980
81. Fishman, N.H., Bronstein, M.H.: Is mediastinoscopy necessary in the evaluation of lung cancer? Ann. Thorac. Surg. *20,* 678 (1975)
82. Fontana, R.S.: Early diagnosis in lung cancer. Editorial. Am. Rev. Resp. Dis. *116,* 399 (1977)
83. Fosburg, R.G., O'Sullivan, M.J., Gibbons, J.A., Oury, J.H.: Positive mediastinoscopy. An ominous finding. Ann. Thorac. Surg. *18,* 346 (1974)
84. Fox, W., Scadding, J.G.: Medical research council comparative trial of surgery and radiotherapy for primary treatment of small celled or oat-celled carcinoma of the bronchus. Lancet *2,* 63 (1973)
85. Franke, H.D., Kunstmann, H.W.: Strahlentherapie des Bronchialkarzinoms. Internist *11,* 338 (1970)
86. Freise, G., Gabler, A., Liebig, S.: Bronchial carcinoma and long-term survival. Thorax *33,* 228 (1978)
87. Freisleben, R.: Funktionelle Kontraindikationen. In: Denck, H., Sighart, H.: Das Bronchuskarzinom heute. Adolf Holzhausen Nfg., Wien 1980
88. Fryjordet, A., Klevmark, B.: Investigation of operability in cases of bronchial carcinoma. Scand. J. Thorac. Cardiovasc. Surg. *5,* 97 (1971)
89. Gabler, A., Liebig, S.: Reoperation for bronchial carcinoma. Thorax *35,* 668 (1980)
90. Gall, W.: Fünfjahresergebnisse (Langzeitergebnisse) nach Lungenresektion wegen Plattenepithelkarzinoms und die Bedeutung dieser Ergebnisse für die Früherkennung. Prax. Pneumol. *30,* 649 (1976)
91. Geddes, D.M., Green, M., Emerson, P.A.: Lung function tests: comparison of reports by physician and computer. Thorax *33,* 257 (1978)
92. Geroulanos, S., Senning, Å.: Indikation und Ergebnisse operativer Therapie beim Bronchuskarzinom. Therapeutische Umschau *35,* 1029 (1978)
93. Ghosh, P., Pakrashi, B.C.: Cardiac dysrhythmias after throracotomy. Brit. Heart J. *34,* 374 (1972)
93a. Giaccone, G., Rocmans, P., Vanderschueren, R.G. (EORTC/NCI Lung Cancer Study Group): Adjuvant surgery after induction chemotherapy in limited disease small cell lung cancer. A randomized prospective study. European Organization for Research on Treatment of Cancer 0845 Netherlands Cancer Institute. Amsterdam, Jan. 1985
94. Gobbel, W.G., Sawyers, J.L., Rhea, W.G.: Experience with palliative resection and irradiation therapy for carcinoma of the lung. J. Thorac. Surg. *53,* 183 (1967)
95. Goldberg, E.M.: Mediastinoscopy in assessment of lung cancer. In: Straus, M.J.: Lung cancer; clinical diagnosis and treatment. Grune & Stratton, New York/San Francisco/London 1979
96. Goldberg, E.M., Glicksmam, A.S., Khan, F.R., Nickon, J.J.: Mediastinoscopy for assessing mediastinal spread in clinical staging of carcinoma of the lung. Cancer *25,* 347 (1970)

97. Goldstraw, P.: Postpneumonectomy empyema. J. Thorac. Cardiovasc. Surg. *79,* 851 (1980)
98. Goldstraw, P.: Prophylaxis of postpneumonectomy empyema. Thorax *35,* 107 (1980)
98a. Goldstraw, P., Harper, P.G., Rocmans, P. (EORTC *Lung Cancer Study Group): Surgery + chemotherapy vs. surgery alone in the treatment of stage I small cell carcinoma of the lung, a randomized prospective study. European Organization for Research on Treatment of Cancer 08843. Amsterdam, Febr. 1984
99. Greco, F.A., Oldham, R.K.: Clinical management of patients with small cell lung cancer. In: Greco, F.A., Oldham, R.K., Bunn, P.A.: Small cell lung cancer. Grune & Stratton, New York 1981
99a. Greene, R.: Radiological studies of thoracic neoplasms. In: Choi, N.C., Grillo, H.C. eds.: Thoracic Oncology. Raven Press, New York 1983
100. Greschuchna, D., Maassen, D.,: Über die intrapulmonalen und mediastinalen Ausbreitungswege des Bronchialkarzinoms. Thoraxchir. *19,* 434 (1971)
101. Greschuchna, D., Maassen, W.: Die lymphogenen Absiedlungswege des Bronchialkarzinoms. Georg Thieme Verlag, Stuttgart 1973
102. Greschuchna, D.: Ergebnisse der operativen Behandlung des kleinzelligen Bronchialkarzinoms. Thoraxchirurgie *26,* 300 (1978)
103. Gütgemann, A., Kreutzberg, B., Lichtenthäler, J., Savic, B.: Ergebnisse und Erfahrungen zum Bronchuskarzinom. Studie über 20 Jahre. Med. Welt *27,* 835 (1976)
104. Guinn, G.A., Tomm, K.E., North, L., Mocega, E.: Clinical staging of primary lung cancer. Chest *64,* 51 (1973)
105. Gutierrez, A.C., Vincent, R.G., Bakshi, S., Takita, H.: Radioisotope scans in the evaluation of metastatic bronchogenic carcinoma. J. Thorac. Cardiovasc. Surg. *69,* 934 (1975)
106. Haas, Ch.E., Lebas, F.X., Choubrac, P.: Les opacités rondes solitaires intra-pulmonaires. Conduite diagnostique et thérapeutique. Le poumon et le coeur *3,* 315 (1977)
107. Hamelmann, H.: Radikale Eingriffe bei ausgedehnten malignen Tumoren im Thoraxbereich. Chirurg. *39,* 109 (1968)
108. Hansen, H.H., Muggia, F.M.: Early detection of bone-marrow invasion in oat cell carcinoma of the lung. N. Engl. J. Med. *284,* 962 (1971)
109. Hansen, H.H.: Management of lung cancer. Med. Clin. North Am. *61,* 979 (1977)
110. Hansen, H.H., Muggia, F.M., Selawry, O.S.: Bone-marrow examination in 100 consecutive patients with bronchogenic carcinoma. Lancet *2,* 443 (1971)
111. Harazim, H., Kaik, G., Kaik, B.: Beitrag zur Klinik und Therapie des Alveolarzellkarzinoms. Pneumologie *148,* 281 (1973)
112. Harley, H.R.S.: Cancer of the lung in women. Thorax *31,* 254 (1976)
113. Harmom, H., Fergus, S., Cole, F.H.: Pneumonectomy: review of 351 cases. Ann. Surg. *183,* 719 (1976)
114. Harms, H., Jüngst, G., Windheim, K.v.: Postoperative Funktionsentwicklung nach Lungenresektion: Frühphase. Pneumologie *147,* 126 (1972)
115. Hartel, W., Lenz, J., Schuster, G., Kohlkapp, E.: Der zentrale Venendruck bei Lungenresektionen. Thoraxchir. *17,* 198 (1969)
116. Harviel, J.D., Mc Namara, J.J., Straehley, C.J.: Surgical treatment of lung cancer in patients over the age of 70 years. J. Thorac. Cardiovasc. Surg. *75,* 802 (1978)
117. Hasse, J.: Zur Chirurgie des Lungenkarzinoms, Editorial. Schweiz. Rundschau Med. (Praxis) *70,* 501 (1981)
118. Hasse, J., Perruchoud, A., Wolff, G., Grädel, E.: Right-to-left atrial shunt in cardiac dislocation following extensive pneumonectomy. Thorac. Cardiovasc. Surgeon *27,* 330 (1979)
119. Hasse, J.: Unpublished data
119a. Hasse, J., Palas, T., Skarvan, K., Grädel, E.: Hybrid ventilation technique – IPPV/HF-Jetventilation – for secondary pulmonary resection at the tracheal bifurcation. Thorac. cardiovasc. Surgeon *32,* Spec. issue I, 82 (1984)
120. Hata, E., Troidl, H., Hasegawa, T.: In-vivo-Untersuchungen der Lymphdrainage. In: Hamelmann, H., Troidl, H.: Behandlung des Bronchialkarzinoms. Georg Thieme, Stuttgart 1981

121. Hattori, S., Matsuda, M., Tateishi, R., Nishihara, H., Horai, T.: Oat-cell carcinoma of the lung. Cancer *30,* 1014 (1972)
122. Hauck, M.: Risiko und Erfolg der Bronchialkarzinom-Chirurgie. Eine statistische Analyse. Inauguraldissertation, Giessen 1977
123. Hecht, A.: Die cytostatische und kombinierte Behandlung des Bronchialkarzinoms. Pneumologie *145,* 158 (1970)
124. Heilmann, H.P., Doppelfeld, E., Fernholz, H.-J., et al.: Ergebnisse der Strahlenbehandlung des Bronchialkarzinoms. Dtsch. med. Wschr. *101,* 1557 (1976)
125. Heindl, W., Zwick, E.: Präoperative pulmokardiale Funktionsbeurteilung bei Patienten mit zu resezierendem Bronchuskarzinom. In: Denck, H., Sighart, H.: Das Bronchuskarzinom heute. Adolf Holzhausen Nfg., Wien 1980
126. Heitzmann, E.R., Proto, A.V., Goldwin, R.L.: The role of computerized tomography in the diagnosis of diseases of the thorax. JAMA *241,* 933 (1979)
127. Henney, J., Ishikawa, S., Jacobs, E.M.: Surgical aspects: overview. In: Muggia, F.M., Rozencweig, M.: Lung cancer (Progress in cancer research and therapy, vol. 11). Raven Press, New York 1979
128. Herfarth, Ch.: Organisation einer interdisziplinären Onkologie aus chirurgischer Sicht. Chirurg. *49,* 529 (1978)
128a. Hermanek, P., Gall, F.P.: Lungentumoren. Kompendium der klinischen Tumorpathologie. Bd. 2 Witzstrock, G., Baden-Baden 1979
129. Herzog, H.: Störungen der Respirationsorgane als Ursache der pulmonalen Hypertonie. Thoraxchir. *14,* 500 (1966)
130. Higgins, G.A.: Use of chemotherapy as an adjuvant to surgery for bronchogenic carcinoma. Cancer *30,* 1383 (1972)
131. Higgins, G.A., Lawton, R., Heilbrunn, A., Keehn, R.J.: Prognostic factors in lung cancer. Surgical aspects. Ann. Thorac. Surg. *7,* 472 (1969)
132. Higgins, G.A., Shields, T.W., Keehn, R.J.: The solitary pulmonary nodule. 10 year follow-up of Veterans Administration Armed Forces cooperative study. Arch. Surg. *110,* 570 (1975)
133. Hilaris, B.S., Martini, N., Batata, M., Beattie, E.J.: Interstitial irradiation for unresectable carcinoma of the lung. Ann. Thorac. Surg. *20,* 491 (1975)
134. Hilton, G.: Present position relating to cancer. Results with radiotherapy alone. Thorax *15,* 17 (1960)
135. Hinson, K.F.W., Miller, A.B., Tall, R.: An assessment of the W.H.O. classification of the histologic type of lung tumors applied to biopsy and resected material. Cancer *35,* 399 (1975)
136. Hoffmann, E., Jünemann, A., Pisa, G.: Ergebnisse beim resezierten Bronchialkarzinom in Abhängigkeit von Lymphknotenbefall und Tumorlokalisation. Bruns Beitr. Klin. Chir. *218,* 518 (1971)
137. Høgsbro, A., Østergaard, L.: Surgery for carcinoma of the lung in patients over 70 years. Scand. J. Thorac. Cardiovasc. Surg. *1,* 197 (1967)
138. Holly, P.C., Hill, L.D., Lawless, P.A., West, T.L.: Cardiac disturbances after pneumonectomy. The value of prophylactic digitalization. Ann. Chir. Gynaecol. *67,* 77 (1978)
139. Hooper, R.G., Beechler, C.R., Johnson, M.C.: Radioisotope scanning in the initial staging of bronchogenic carcinoma. Am. Rev. Resp. Dis. *118,* 279 (1978)
140. Hoppe, R.: 20 000mal Verdacht auf Lungenkrebs. Prax. Pneumol. *31,* 872 (1977)
141. Horn, J., Kauffmann, G.W.: Zur gesundheitlichen Überwachung und Rehabilitation operierter Lungenkrebskranker im Berliner Raum. Z. Erkr. Atm. Org. *147,* 219 (1977)
142. Huber, F.B.: Die Klinik des Adenokarzinoms der Bronchien und die operativen Spätergebnisse. Thoraxchir. *17,* 334 (1969)
143. Huber, H., Rieche, K.: Kombinierte Behandlungsmodalitäten beim Bronchuskarzinom. In: Huber, H., Senn, H., Falkensammler, M., Hrsg.: Adjuvante zytostatische Therapie. Springer, Berlin/Heidelberg/New York 1978
144. Hutchinson, C.M., Mills, N.L.: The selection of patients with bronchogenic carcinoma for mediastinoscopy. J. Thorac. Cardiovasc. Surg. *71,* 768 (1976)
145. Huth, J.H., Diwok, K.: Intra- und postoperative Komplikationen durch Eingriffe an der Lunge. Z. Erkrank. Atm. Org. *151,* 231 (1978)

146. Hyde, L.H., Wolf, J., McCracken, S., Yesner, R.: Natural course of inoperable lung cancer. Chest *64,* 309 (1973)
147. Ikeda, S.: Flexible bronchofiberscope. Ann. Otol. Rhinol. Laryngol. *79,* 916 (1970)
148. Ioachim, H.L.: Present trends in lung cancer. In: Thurlbeck, W.M. ed.: The lung, structure, function and disease. Williams and Wilkins, Baltimore 1978.
149. Jackman, R.J., Good, C.A., Clagett, O.T., Woolner, L.B.: Survival rates in peripheral bronchogenic carcinomas up to four cm in diameter presenting as solitary pulmonary nodules. J. Thorac. Cardiovasc. Surg. *57,* 1 (1969)
150. James, E.C., Schuchmann, G.F., Hall, R.V., Patterson, J.R., Gillespie, J.T., Gomez, A.C.: Preferred surgical treatment for alveolar carcinoma. Ann. Thorac. Surg. *22,* 157 (1976)
151. Jamieson, M.P.G., Walbaum, P.R., McCormack, R.J.M.: Surgical management of bronchial carcinoma invading the chest wall. Thorax *34,* 612 (1979)
152. Jenny, H.: Histologie, Tumorstadium und Lebenserwartung beim Bronchialkarzinom. Thoraxchir. *19,* 244 (1971)
153. Jenny, H., Buchenberger, R.: Histologie, Tumorstadium und Lebenserwartung beim Bronchuskarzinom. Langenb. Arch. *325,* 522 (1969)
154. Jensik, R.J., Faber, L.P., Milloy, F.J., Amato, J.J.: Sleeve lobectomy for carcinoma. A ten-year experience. J. Thorac. Cardiovasc. Surg. *64,* 400 (1972)
155. Jensik, R.J.: Die Berechtigung zur parenchymsparenden Resektion. In: Hamelmann, H., Troidl, H.: Behandlung des Bronchialkarzinoms. Georg Thieme, Stuttgart 1981
156. Jezek V.: Pulmonary haemodynamics in bronchogenic cancer before and after lung resection. Prog. Resp. Res. *5,* 237 (1970)
157. Johansson, L., Westerholm, C.J., Wranne, B.: Central circulatory function early after pulmonary surgery. Scand. J. Thorac. Cardiovasc. Surg. *4,* 107 (1970)
158. Johnson, R.R.J.: Radiotherapy – primary and/or adjuvant modality. In: Perspectives in Lung Cancer. Karger, Basel 1977
159. Jolly, Ph.C., Hill, L.D., Lawless, P.A., West, Th.L.: Parasternal mediastinotomy and mediastinoscopy. J. Thorac. Cardiovasc. Surg. *66,* 549 (1973)
160. Jones, J.C., Robinson, J.L., Meyer, B.W., Motley, H.L.: Primary carcinoma of the lung. A follow-up study including pulmonary function studies of long-term survivors. J. Thorac. Cardiovasc. Surg. *39,* 144 (1960)
161. Jost, R.G., Stagel, S.S., Stanley, R.J., Levitt, R.G.: Computed tomography of the thorax. Radiology *126,* 125 (1978)
162. Kaiser, D.: Diagnostik peripher gelegener Bronchialkarzinome. Therapiewoche *29,* 7198 (1979)
163. Kaiser, D.: Die Abklärung der lokalen Operabilität des Bronchialkarzinoms. Therapiewoche *29,* 7203 (1979)
164. Kaiser, D.: Die operative Behandlung des Bronchialkarzinoms. Therapiewoche *29,* 7213 (1979)
165. Kaplan, E.D., Meier, P.: Nonparametric estimation from incomplete observations. Am. Statist. Assoc. J. *53,* 457 (1958)
166. Karrer, K., Pridun, N., Denck, H., Sighart, H.: Polychemotherapie bei Patienten nach radikaler Operation wegen Bronchuskarzinom. Oesterr. Zschr. Onkologie *3,* 127 (1976)
167. Karrer, K.: Zytostatische Adjuvanstherapie beim Bronchialkarzinom. In: Huber, H., Senn, H., Falkensammler, M., Hrsg.: Adjuvante zytostatische Chemotherapie. Springer, Berlin/Heidelberg/New York 1978
168. Katsuki, H., Shimada, H., Koyama, A., Okita, M., Yamaguchi, Y.: Long-term intermitted adjuvant chemotherapy for primary, resected lung cancer. J. Thorac. Cardiovasc. Surg. *70,* 590 (1975)
169. Keller, R.: Die Auswirkungen chronisch obstruktiver Atemwegserkrankungen auf das Herz-Kreislauf-System. Therapeutische Umschau *34,* 172 (1977)
170. Kerr, W.F.: Late-onset post-pneumonectomy empyema. Thorax *32,* 149 (1977)
171. Kirsh, M.M., Prior, M., Gago, O., Moores, W.Y., Kahn, D.R., Pellegrini, R.V., Sloan, H.: The effect of histological cell type on the prognosis of patients with bronchogenic carcinoma. Ann. Thorac. Surg. *13,* 303 (1972)
172. Kirsh, M.M., Rotman, H., Behrendt, D.M., Orringer, M.B., Sloan, H.: Complications of pulmonary resection. Ann. Thorac. Surg. *20,* 215 (1975)

173. Kirsh, M.M., Rotman, H., Argenta, L., Bove, E., Cimmino, V., Tashian, J., Ferguson, P., Sloan, H.: Carcinoma of the lung: Results of treatment over ten years. Ann. Thorac. Surg. *21,* 371 (1976)
174. Kodras, B., Heindel, W.: Postoperatives Management nach Lungenresektionen. In: Denck, H., Sighart, H.: Das Bronchuskarzinom heute. Adolf Holzhausen Nfg., Wien 1980
174a. König, R., van Kaick, G., Vogt-Moykopf, I.: Was leistet die Computertomographie für die Beurteilung bronchopulmonaler und mediastinaler Lymphknoten beim Bronchialkarzinom. Prax. Klin. Pneumol. *38,* 438 (1984)
175. Kraft-Kinz, J., Eder, J., Kronberger, L., List, W.: Erfahrungen mit der chirurgischen Behandlung von Lungentumoren. Thoraxchirurgie *18,* 9 (1970)
176. Krause, F.: Spätergebnisse operativer Behandlung des bronchogenen Plattenepithel-Karzinoms. Prax. Pneumol. *31,* 202 (1977)
177. Kreyberg, L.: Histological typing of lung tumors. World Health Organization, Geneva 1967
178. Krokowski, E.: Befindet sich die kurative Krebstherapie in der Sackgasse? Dtsch. med. Wschr. *104,* 326 (1979)
179. Kurpat, D., Anstett, K.: Arbeitsunfähigkeit, Invalidisierung und berufliche Rehabilitation nach Operation wegen Bronchialkarzinom. Z. Erkrankg. Atm. Org. *147,* 223 (1977)
180. Kurpat, D., Bredel, P., Metzger, B.: Keilresektion beim Bronchialkarzinom. Z. Erkrankg. Atm. Org. *155,* 41 (1980)
181. Kutschera, W.: Ergebnisse der erweiterten Lungenresektion beim Bronchuskarzinom. Thoraxchir. *19,* 461 (1971)
182. Kutschera, W.: Bronchuskarzinom, Abhängigkeit des Operationserfolges. Thoraxchir. *24,* 164 (1976)
183. Kutschera, W., Schnetzer, J.: Kombinierte operative und cytostatische Behandlung des Bronchialcarcinoms. Pneumologie *145,* 139 (1970)
184. Kutschera, W.: Symptomatik und Prognose des Bronchuskarzinoms. In: Denck, H., Sighart, H.: Das Bronchuskarzinom heute. Adolf Holzhausen Nfg., Wien 1980
185. Lacquet, L.K.: La valeur de la médiastinoscopie dans le traitement chirurgical du cancer pulmonaire. Ann. Chir. Thorac. Cardiovasc. *15,* 323 (1976)
186. Lacquet, L.K., Mertens, A., Van Kleef, J., Jongerius, C.: Mediastinoscopy and bronchial carcinoma: experience with 600 mediastinoscopies. Thorax *30,* 141 (1975)
186a. Laros, C.D.: Lung function data on 123 persons followed up for 20 years after total pneumonectomy. Respiration *43,* 81 (1982)
187. Latarjet, M., Bes, J.: The surgical treatment of primary bronchopulmonary cancer. In: Surgical Oncology – Current Problems of Surgery. Huber, Bern 1970
188. Laufman, H.: Nosocomial infection complicating intrathoracic surgery. In Cordell, A.R., Ellison, R.G., eds.: Complications of intrathoracic surgery. Little, Brown & Company, Boston 1979
189. Laurenzi, G.A., Marks, C.E., Peabody, J.W., Ross, J.C., Utz, J.P., Young, R.C., Cugell, D.W.: Diagnostic mediastinoscopy. Am. Rev. Respir. Dis. *105,* 487 (1972)
190. Lawrence, G.H., Walker, J.H., Pinkers, L.: Extended resection of bronchogenic carcinoma. New Engl. J. Medicine *263,* 615 (1960)
191. Lee, R.E.: Radiotherapy for lung cancer. In: Straus, M.J.: Lung cancer; clinical diagnosis and treatment. Grune & Stratton, New York/San Francisco/London 1977
192. Lesch, R.: Das Bronchialkarzinom. Nomenklatur–Morphologie–Präneoplasien. Therapiewoche *29,* 7157 (1979)
193. Liebig, S., Gabler, A., Raffenberg, M.: Standardisierte antibiotische Therapie in der großen Lungenchirurgie. Prax. Pneumol. *33,* 548 (1979)
194. Line, D.H., Deeley, T.J.: The necropsy findings in carcinoma of the bronchus. Brit. J. Dis. Chest *65,* 238 (1971)
195. Livingston, R.B.; Trauth, C.J., Greenstreet, R.L.: Small cell carcinoma: clinical manifestations and behavior with treatment. In: Greco, F.A., Oldham, R.K., Bunn, P.A.: Small cell lung cancer. Grune & Stratton, New York 1981
196a. Lockwood, P.: The principles of predicting the risk of postthoracotomy functional-related complications in bronchial carcinoma. Respiration *30,* 329 (1973)
196b. Lockwood, P.: The relationship between preoperative lung function test results and postoperative complications in carcinoma of the bronchus. Respiration *30,* 105 (1973)

197. Lockwood, P.: Airway obstruction in patients with carcinoma of the bronchus. Respiration *36,* 50 (1978)

197a. Ludwig Lung Cancer Study group: Search for the possible role of 'immunotherapy' in operable bronchial non-small cell carcinoma (stage I and II): A phase I study with *Corynebacterium* parvum intrapleurally. Cancer Immunol. Immunther. *4,* 69 (1978)

198. Lüdeke, H.: Diagnostik des Bronchialkarzinoms. Langenbecks Arch. *325,* 490 (1969)

199. Lukeman, J.M.: What is lung cancer? In: Perspectives in Lung Cancer. Karger, Basel 1977

200. Lukeman, J.M., Wilson, R.A., Samuel, R.F.: Cytologic and histologic correlation of lung tumors. In: Muggia, F.M., Rozencweig, M.: Lung cancer (Progress in cancer research and therapy, vol. 11). Raven Press, New York 1979

201. Luomanen, K.J., Watson, W.L.: Autopsy findings. In: Watson, W.L. (ed.): Lung cancer, a study of five thousand Memorial Hospital cases. Mosby, St. Louis 1968

202. Maassen, W., Greschuchna, D.: Allgemeine und spezielle Ergebnisse der Mediastinoskopie (2500) unter besonderer Berücksichtigung des Bronchialkarzinoms. Thoraxchir. *19,* 289 (1971)

203. Maassen, W.: Ergebnisse und Bedeutung der Mediastinoskopie und anderer bioptischer Verfahren. Springer, Heidelberg 1976

204. Mac Hale, S.J.: Carcinoma of the bronchus. In: Smith, R.E. and Williams, W.G.: Surgery of the lung. Butterworth, London 1974

205. Mack, D., Mallinckrodt, G. v., Brandmair, W., Dittler, H.J., Harlacher, A.: Ergebnisse der Behandlung des operierten Bronchuscarzinoms und des nicht operierten kleinzellig-anaplastischen Carcinoms. Langenbecks Arch. Chir. *351,* 77 (1980)

206. Mandelbaum, I., Williams, S.D., Hornback, B., Joe, M.B., Einhorn, L.H.: Combined therapy for small cell undifferentiated carcinoma of the lung. J. Thorac. Cardiovasc. Surg. *76,* 292 (1978)

207. Marsh, B.R., Frost, J.K., Erozan, Y.S., Carter, D.: Fiberbronchoscopy. In: Straus, M.J.: Lung cancer. Grune & Stratton, New York 1977

208. Martini, N., Melamed, M.R.: Multiple primary lung cancers. J. Thorac. Cardiovasc. Surg. *70,* 606 (1975)

209. Matthes, Th., Widow, W., Berndt, H., Wildner, G.P., Ritzow, H., Peek, U., Marx, G., Wolf, M., Klein, K.: 20jährige Erfahrungen in der Behandlung des Bronchialkarzinoms aus chirurgischer Sicht. Teil I: Arch. Geschwulstforsch. *34,* 227 (1969) Teil II: Arch. Geschwulstforsch. *34,* 336 (1969)

210. Matthews, M.J., Kanhouwa, S., Pickren, J., Robinette, D.: Frequency of residual and metastatic tumor in patients undergoing curative surgical resection for lung cancer. Cancer Chemother. Rep. *4,* 63 (1973)

211. Matthews, M.J., Gordon, Ph.R.: Morphology of pulmonary and pleural malignancies. In: Straus, M.J., (ed.): Lung cancer. Grune & Stratton, New York 1977

212. Matthews, M.J.: Effects of therapy on the morphology and behavior of small cell carcinoma of the lung – a clinicopathologic study. In: Muggia, F.M., M. Rozencweig: Lung cancer. Raven Press, New York 1979

213. Matthews, M.J., Pickren, J., Kanhouwa, S.: Who has occult metastases? In: Perspectives in lung cancer. Karger, Basel 1977

214. Matthys, H.: Das Bronchuskarzinom. Therapiewoche *29,* 7144 (1979)

215. McNeill, Th.M., Chamberlain, J.M.: Diagnostic anterior mediastinotomy. Ann. Thorac. Surg. *2,* 532 (1966)

216. Mégevand, R., Brand, U., Huber, O., Spilopoulus, A.: Survie des cancers bronchopulmonaires opérés. Schweiz. med. Wschr. *109,* 851 (1979)

217. Melamed, M.R.: Pathology. In: Watson, W.L. (ed.): Lung cancer, a study of five thousand Memorial Hospital cases. Mosby, St. Louis 1968

218. Melamed, M.R., Cahan, W.G.: Cytology. In: Watson, W.L. (ed.): Lung cancer, a study of five thousand Memorial Hospital cases. Mosby, St. Louis 1968

219. Merrick, D.K., Carr, D.T., Payne, W.S., Woolner, L.B.: Multiple primary cancer of the lung. Geriatrics *27,* 71 (1972)

220. Meyers, G., Lembeck, L., O'Kane, H., Baue, A.E.: Changes in functional residual capacity of the lung after operation. Arch. Surg. *110,* 576 (1975)

221. Miller, W.E.: Roentgenographic manifestations of lung cancer. In: Straus, M.J.: Lung cancer; clinical diagnosis and treatment. Grune & Stratton, New York/San Francisco/London 1977
222. Minna, J.D., Brereton, H.D., Cohen, M.H., Ihde, D.C., Bunn, P.A., Shackney, S.E., Fossieck, B.E., Matthews, M.J.: The treatment of small cell carcinoma of the lung: prospects for cure. In: Muggia, F., Rozencweig, M. eds.: Lung cancer: Progress in therapeutic research. Raven Press, New York 1979
223. Mintzer, R.A., Malave, S.R., Neiman, H.C., Michaelis, L.L., Vanecke, R.M., Sanders, J.H.: Computed vs. conventional tomography in evaluation of primary and secondary neoplasms. Radiology *132,* 653 (1979)
224. Mittman, Ch., Bruderman, I.: Lung cancer: to operate or not? Am. Rev. Resp. Dis. *116,* 477 (1977)
225. Mosberg, W.H.: Twelve-year "cure" of lung cancer with metastasis to the brain. JAMA *235,* 2745 (1976)
226. Mossberg, B., Björk, V.O., Holmgren, A.: Working capacity and cardiopulmonary function after extensive lung resections. Scand. J. Thorac. Cardiovasc. Surg. *10,* 247 (1976)
227. Mountain, C.F.: Biologic, physiologic and technical determinants in surgical therapy for lung cancer. In: Straus, M.J.: Lung Cancer; clinical diagnosis and treatment. Grune & Stratton, New York/San Francisco/London 1977
228. Mountain, C.F.: A surgeon's insight into tumor behaviour. In: Perspectives in lung cancer. Karger, Basel 1977
229. Mountain, C.F., Hermes, K.E.: Management implications of surgival staging studies. In: Muggia, F.M., Rozencweig, M.: Lung cancer (Progress in cancer research and therapy, vol. 11). Raven Press, New York 1979
230. Mountain, C.F., Carr, D.T., Anderson, W.A.D.: A system for the clinical staging of lung cancer. Am. J. Roentgenol. Radium. Ther. Nucl. Med. *120,* 130 (1974)
231. Mountain, C.F.: Surgical therapy. In Fishman, A.P.: Pulmonary diseases and disorders. Ch. 130. Mac Graw-Hill, New York 1980
232. Muggia, F.M., Hansen, H.H., Chervu, L.R.: Diagnosis in metastatic sites. In: Straus, M.J.: Lung Cancer; clinical diagnosis and treatment. Grune & Stratton, New York/San Francisco/London 1977
233. Muhar, F., Kaik, G., Raber, A., Scheiblechner, H.: Funktionelle Spätergebnisse nach Lungenresektion. Pneumologie *147,* 145 (1972)
234. Naef, A.P.: Tracheobronchialresektion. Thoraxchir. *20,* 283 (1972)
235. Naef, A.P.: New techniques in the surgical treatment of lung cancer. In: Straus, M.J.: Lung cancer; clinical diagnosis and treatment. Grune & Stratton, New York/San Francisco/London 1977
236. Naef, A.P.: La chirurgie du cancer bronchique. Schweiz. med. Wschr. *109,* 816 (1979)
237. Naruke, T., Yoneyama, T., Ogata, T., Suemasu, K.: Bronchoplastic procedures for lung cancer. J. Thorac. Cardiovasc. Surg. *75,* 92 (1977)
238. Navratil, M., Koval, Z., Lichtenberg, J., Mostecky, H.: Postoperative Funktionsentwicklung bei Patienten mit Bronchialcarcinom nach Lungenresektion. Lanzeitprognose. Pneumologie *147,* 136 (1972)
239. Neumann, M.: Nachsorge nach operiertem Lungenkarzinom. In: Denck, H., Sighart, H.: Das Bronchuskarzinom heute. Adolf Holzhausen Nfg., Wien 1980
240. Niederle, N., Seeber, S., Konietzko, N., Schmidt, C.G.: Kombinierte Chemo- und Radiotherapie (ACO II plus RT) des inoperablen kleinzelligen und anaplastisch-großzelligen Bronchialkarzinoms. Prax. Pneumol. *34,* 533 (1980)
241. Nohl, H.C.: A three-year follow-up of classified cases of bronchogenic carcinoma after resection. Thorax *15,* 11 (1960)
242. Nohl, H.C.: The long-term survival of patients with lung cancer treated surgically after selection by mediastinoscopy. Thoracic and Cardiovasc. Surgeon *28,* 158 (1980)
243. Nolte, D.: Auswirkungen der operativen Behandlung des Bronchialcarcinoms auf die Atemmechanik. Pneumonologie *145,* 170 (1971)
244. Nowicki, J.: Funktionelle und soziale Spätergebnisse nach Lungenoperationen. Z. Erkrank. Atm. Org. *148,* 204 (1977)
245. Oesch, A., Nachbur, B., Senn, A.: Ergebnisse der Resektionsbehandlung des Bronchial-

karzinoms bei einem mediastinoskopisch selektionierten Krankengut. Thoraxchir. *19,* 444 (1971)

246. Oeser, H.: Aspekte der röntgenologischen Früherkennung des Lungenkrebses. Prax. Pneumol. *30,* 1 (1976)
247. Olbert, F.: Lungenkrebs: Früherkennung und Angiographie. In: Denck, H., Sighart, H.: Das Bronchuskarzinom heute. Adolf Holzhausens Nachf. Wien 1979
248. Olsen, G.N., Block, A.J., Swenson, E.W., Castle, J.R., Wynne, J.W.: Pulmonary function evaluation of the lung resection candidate: a prospective study. Am. Rev. Resp. Dis. *111,* 379 (1975)
249. Overholt, R.H., Neptune, W.B., Ashraf, M.M.: Primary cancer of the lung. Ann. Thorac. Surg. *20,* 511 (1975)
250. Pancoast, H.K.: Superior pulmonary sulcus tumor. J.A.M.A. *99,* 1391 (1932)
251. Paneth, M.: Behandlung des Bronchial-Karzinoms mit Manschettenresektion. Thoraxchir. *20,* 285 (1972)
252. Paris, F., Tarazona, V., Blasco, E., Canto, A., Casillas, M., Pastor, J.: Mediastinoscopy in the surgical management of lung carcinoma. Thorax *30,* 146 (1975)
253. Paulson, D.L.: A philosophy of treatment of bronchogenic carcinoma. Ann. Thorac. Surg. *5,* 289 (1968)

253a. Paulson, D.L.: Management of superior sulcus carcinomas, in Choi, N.C., H.C. Grillo: Thoracic Oncology. Raven Press, New York 1983

254. Paulson, D.L., Reisch, J.S.: Long term survival after resection for bronchogenic carcinoma. Ann. Surg. *184,* 324 (1976)
255. Paulson, D.L., Urschel, H.C.: Selectivity in the surgical treatment of bronchogenic carcinoma. J. Thorac. Cardiovasc. Surg. *62,* 554 (1971)
256. Paulson, D.L., Urschel, H.C., McNamara, J.J., Shaw, R.R.: Bronchoplastic procedures for bronchogenic carcinoma. J. Thorac. Cardiovasc. Surg. *59,* 38 (1970)
257. Payne, W.S.: Frühentdeckung des Lungenkarzinoms. Ein Zwischenbericht. In: Hamelmann H., Troidl, J.: Behandlung des Bronchialkarzinoms. Georg Thieme Verlag, Stuttgart 1981
258. Payne, C.R., Stovin, P., Barker, V., Mc Vittie, S., Stark, J.E.: Diagnostic accuracy of cytology and biopsy in primary bronchial carcinoma. Thorax *34,* 294 (1979)
259. Peace, P.K., Price, J.L.: Preoperative tomographic assessment of the mediastinum in bronchial carcinoma. Thorax *28,* 367 (1973)
260. Pearson, F.G.: An evaluation of mediastinoscopy in the management of presumably operable bronchial carcinoma. J. Thorac. Cardiovasc. Surg. *55,* 617 (1968)
261. Pearson, F.G.: Assessment of resectability and operability in bronchial carcinoma. In: Murray, G.F., ed.: Cancer of the lung. Stratton, New York/London 1974
262. Pearson, F.G., Nelems, J.M., Henderson, R.D.: The role of mediastinoscopy in the selection of treatment for bronchial carcinoma with involvement of superior mediastinal lymph nodes. J. Thorac. Cardiovasc. Surg. *18,* 433 (1972)
263. Pecora, D.V., Brook, R.: Evaluation of cardiopulmonary reserve in candidates for chest surgery. J. Thorac. Cardiovasc. Surg. *44,* 60 (1962)
264. Perruchoud, A., Meili, U., Hasse, J., Grädel, E., Herzog, H.: Lungenfunktionsprüfung und Untersuchung der Hämodynamik im kleinen Kreislauf bei Bronchialkarzinom. Schweiz. med. Wschr. *109,* 832 (1979)
265. Pertovich, Z., Ohanian, M., Cox, J.: Clinical research on the treatment of locally advanced lung cancer. Final report of VALG protocol 13 limited. Cancer *42,* 1129 (1978)
266. Peterfy, A., Calabrese, E.: Mechanical and conventional manual sutures of the bronchial stump. Scand. J. Thor. Cardiovasc. Surg. *13,* 87 (1979)
267. Peters, R.M., Clausen, J.L., Tisi, G.M.: Extending resectibility for carcinoma of the lung in patients with impaired pulmonary function. Ann. Thorac. Surg. *26,* 250 (1978)
268. Peto, R., Pike, M.C., Armitage, P., Breslow, N.E., Cox, D.R., Howard, S.V., Mantel, N., McPershon, K., Peto, J., Smith, P.G.: Design and analysis of randomized clinical trials requiring prolonged observation of each patient. I. Introduction and design. Br. J. Cancer *34,* 585 (1976) II. Analysis and examples. Br. J. Cancer *35,* 1 (1977)
269. Pilchmaier, H., Speisberg, E.: Organerhaltende Operation des Bronchuscarcinoms. Langenbecks Arch. Chir. *328,* 221 (1971)

270. Pool, J.L., Conte, A.J.: Surgical procedures for diagnosis. In: Watson, W.L. (ed.): Lung cancer, a study of five thousand Memorial Hospital cases. Mosby, St. Louis 1968
271. Price-Thomas, C.: Lobectomy with sleeve resection. Thorax *15*, 9 (1960)
272. Pridun, N.: Sicherung der Diagnose beim Lungenkrebs. In: Denck, H., Sighart, H.: Das Bronchuskarzinom heute. Adolf Holzhausen Nfg., Wien 1980
273. Ramsey, H.E., Cahan, W.G., Beattie, E.J., Humphrey, Ch.: The importance of radical lobectomy in lung cancer. J. Thorac. Vardiovasc. Surg. *58*, 225 (1969)
274. Rasker, J.J., Beekhuis, H., Van de Wal, A.M., Homan van der Heide, J.N., Woldring, M.G.: Cobalt-57-bleomycin scanning of hila and mediastinum in patients with bronchial carcinoma: a prospective study. Thorax *31*, 641 (1976)
275. Rees, G.M., Paneth, M.: Lobectomy with sleeve resection in the treatment of bronchial tumours. Thorax *25*, 160 (1970)
276. Robinson, C.L.N., Burkell, C.C.: Radical versus simple resection for lung neoplasm. Brit. J. Dis. Chest *64*, 226 (1970)
277. Rodescu, D.: Lung Cancer. Med. Clin. North Am. *61*, 1205 (1977)
278. Ross, W.M.: How to deal with bronchogenic carcinoma in the elderly. Geriatrics *31*, 107 (1976)
279. Rossetti, M.: Bewährtes und Problematisches in der Chirurgie des Bronchus-Carcinoms. Aktuelle Chir. *8*, 17 (1973)
280. Rubinstein, I., Baum, G.L., Kalter, Y., Pauzner, Y., Lieberman, Y., Bubis, J.J.: The influence of cell type and lymph node metastases on survival of patients with carcinoma of the lung undergoing thoracotomy. Am. Rev. Resp. Dis. *119*, 253 (1979)
281. Ruckdeschel, J.C., Codish, S.D., Stranahan, A., Mc Kneally, M.F.: Postoperative empyema improves survival in lung cancer. N. Engl. J. Med. *287*, 1013 (1972)
282. Rühle, K.H.: Pneumologisch-internistische Diagnostik des Bronchialkarzinoms. Therapiewoche *29*, 7186 (1979)
283. Rupprecht, H., Bartel, M.: Die Mediastinoskopie in der präoperativen Beurteilung der Operabilität des Bronchialkarzinoms. Z. Erkrank. Atm. Org. *146*, 43 (1976)
284. Salazar, O.M.: Tumor control and radiation toxicity in the treatment of lung cancer. In: Muggia, F.M., Rozencweig, M.R.: Lung cancer. Raven Press, New York 1979
285. Salzer, G.: Klinische Überlegungen zur Histologie des Bronchuskarzinoms. Thoraxchirurgie *15*, 121 (1967)
286. Salzer, G.: Stadieneinteilung des Bronchuskarzinoms. In: Denck H., Sighart, H.: Das Bronchuskarzinom heute. Adolf Holzhausen Nfg. Wien 1980
287. Salzer, G.: Klinischer Versuch zur Verbesserung des Schicksals „Radikaloperierter“ Bronchuskarzinom-Patienten. Z. Erkrank. Atm. Org. *142*, 127 (1975)
288. Salzer, G.: Die Chirurgie der malignen Lungengeschwülste. Chirurg *41*, 289 (1970)
289. Schickedanz, H., Völkner, E.: Der pulmonale Blutdruck in der Pathophysiologie der Lungenresektionsbehandlung. Teil I. Normalwerte, lungenchirurgische Erkrankungen, Operationsletalität. Z. Erkrank. Atm. Org. *145*, 406 (1976) Teil II: Bronchialkarzinom und Lungentuberkulose. Z. Erkrank. Atm. Org. *145*, 415 (1976) Teil III: Prä- und postoperative Untersuchungen Z. Erkrank. Atm. Org. *145*, 422 (1976)
290. Schilling, J.A.: Pulmonary resection and sequelae of thoracic surgery. In: Fenn, W.O., Rahn, H.: Handbook of Physiology, Section 3, Vol. II. American Physiological Society, Washington D.C. 1965
291. Schoen, H.R., Stöhr, U.: Fünfjahresheilung nach Lungenresektion wegen Bronchuskarzinom. Thoraxchir. *19*, 429 (1971)
292. Schulte, H.D., Irlich, G., Wassner, U.J.: Reinterventionen beim Bronchialcarcinom. Langenbecks Arch. *342*, 219 (1976)
293. Schulte, H.D., Jünemann, A.: Behandlungsergebnisse nach Wiedereingriffen beim Bronchialcarcinom. Pneumologie *145*, 150 (1970)
294. Sealy, W.C.: Nonmetastatic extrapulmonary manifestations of carcinoma of the lung. In: Murray, G.F., ed.; Cancer of the lung. Stratton, New York/London 1974
295. Sealy, W.C.: Mediastinoscopy. Ann. Thorac. Surg. *18*, 433 (1974)
296. Seeber, S.: Zur internistischen Therapie des Bronchialkarzinoms. In: Fetzer, J., Füllenbach, D., Gabel, H.: Adriamycin. 2. Bd. Solide Tumoren, Hämoblastosen. Kehrer, Freiburg i. Br. 1978

297. Sensening, D.M., Rossi, N.P., Ehrenhaft, J.L.: Results of the surgical treatment of bronchogenic carcinoma. Surg. Gyn. Obstet. *116,* 279 (1963)
298. Shackney, S.E., Straus, M.J., Bunn, P.A.: The growth characteristics of small cell carcinoma of the lung. In: Greco, F.A., Oldham, R.K., Bunn, P.A.: Small cell lung cancer. Grune & Stratton, New York/London 1981
299. Shaker, I.J., McGee, Z.A., Bender, H.W.: Complications of antibiotic therapy. In: Cordell, A.R., Ellison, R.G.: Complications of intrathoracic surgery. Little, Brown & Company, Boston 1979
300. Shaw, K.M., Luke, D.A.: Lobectomy with sleeve-resection of the bronchus for malignant disease and the influence of the suture material used for bronchial repair. Thorac. Cardiovasc. Surgeon *27,* 325 (1979)
301. Sherman, R.S., Philips, S.J.: Radiologic diagnosis of pulmonary neoplasms. In: Watson, W.L. (ed.): Lung cancer, a study of five thousand Memorial Hospital cases. Mosby, St. Louis 1968
302. Shields, Th.W.: Thoughts concerning the management of patients with carcinoma of the lung. In: Perspectives of lung cancer. Karger, Basel 1977
303. Shields, Th.W., Ujiki, G.T.: Digitalization for prevention of arrhythmias following pulmonary surgery. Surg. Gyn. Obstet. *126,* 743 (1968)
304. Shields, Th.W., Higgins, G.D., Keehn, R.J.: Factors influencing survival after resection for bronchial carcinoma. J. Thorac. Cardiovasc. Surg. *64,* 391 (1972)
305. Shields, Th.W.: Diskussionsbeitrag. 7th Annual Meeting, Society of Thoracic Surgeons, Dallas, Texas, Jan. 1971. Ann. Thorac. Surg. *12,* 382 (1971)
306. Shields, Th.W., Yee, J., Conn, J.H., Robinette, C.D.: Relationship of cell type and lymph node metastasis to survival after resection of bronchial carcinoma. Ann. Thorac. Surg. *20,* 501 (1975)
307. Shore, D.B., Paneth, M.: Survival after resection of small cell carcinoma of the bronchus. Thorax *35,* 819 (1980)
308. Sighart, H.: Die Früherkennung des Lungenkrebses aus klinischer Sicht. In: Denck, H., Sighart, H.: Das Bronchuskarzinom heute. Adolf Holzhausen Nfg., Wien 1980
309. Silver, A.W., Espinas, E.E., Byron, F.X.: The fate of the postresection space. Ann. Thorac. Surg. *2,* 311 (1966)
310. Slack, N.H.: Bronchogenic carcinoma: nitrogen mustard as a surgical adjuvant and factors influencing carcinoma. Cancer *25,* 987 (1970)
311. Slack, N.H., Chamberlain, A., Bross, I.D.J.: Predicting survival following surgery for bronchogenic carcinoma. Chest *62,* 433 (1972)
312. Smith, D.E., Karish, A.F., Chapman, J.P.: Healing of the bronchial stump after pulmonary resection. J. Thorac. Cardiovasc. Surg. *46,* 548 (1963)
313. Smith, R.A.: Preoperative assessment, techniques and results of surgery for bronchial carcinoma. In: Smith, R.E. and Williams, W.G.: Surgery of the lung. Butterworth, London 1974
314. Smith, R.A.: The results of raising the resectability rate in operations for lung carcinoma. J. Thorac. Cardiovasc. Surg. *48,* 418 (1964)
315. Smith, R.A.: The importance of mediastinal lymph node invasion by pulmonary carcinoma in selection of patients for resection. Ann. Thorac. Surg. *25,* 5 (1978)
316. Sobin, L.H.: The WHO histological classification of lung tumors. In: Muggia, F.M., Rozencweig, M.: Lung cancer (Progress in cancer research and therapy, vol. 11): Raven Press, New York 1979
316a. Sobin, L.H., Yesner, R.: Histologic typing of lung tumors. In: World Health Organization: International Histological Classification of Tumors. Geneva 1981
317. Sommerwerck, D.: Ökonomische Teilresektion beim peripheren Bronchialkarzinom. Prax. Pneumol. *24,* 225 (1970)
318. Soorae, A.S., Smith, R.A.: Tumour size as a prognostic factor after resection for lung carcinoma. Thorax *32,* 19 (1977)
319. Soorae, A.S.: Staged bilateral lobectomy for synchronous bilateral squamous cell carcinoma of the lung. Thorax *33,* 511 (1978)
320. Sorensen, H.R.: Die Bedeutung bronchialplastischer Eingriffe für die Therapie des Bronchial-Karzinoms. Thoraxchir. *20,* 274 (1972)

321. Specht, G.: Aktuelle Fragen der chirurgischen Diagnostik und chirurgischen Behandlung des Bronchialcarcinoms. Internist *11,* 331 (1970)
322. Spencer, H.: Pathology of the lung. 3rd Ed., Vol. 11. Pergamon Press, Oxford 1977
323. Spieler, P., Joder, P.: Bronchialzytologie – Bedeutung verschiedener Methoden zur Erfassung primärer Lungenkarzinome. Schweiz. med. Wschr. *109,* 824 (1979)
324. Spjut, H.J., Mateo, L.E.: Recurrent and metastatic carcinoma in surgically treated carcinoma of the lung. Cancer *18,* 1462 (1965)
325. Stafford, E.G., Clagett, O.T.: Post pneumonectomy empyema: neomycin-instillation and definitive closure. J. Thorac. Cardiovasc. Surg. *63,* 771 (1972)
326. Stanek, V., Widimsky, J., Hurych, J., Petrikova, J.: Pressure, flow and volume changes during exercise within pulmonary vascular bed in patients after pneumonectomy. Clin. Sci. *37,* 11 (1969)
327. Stanford, W., Spivey, Ch.G., Larsen, G.L., Alexander, J.A.: Results and treatment of primary carcinoma of the lung. Analysis of 3000 cases. J. Thorac. Cardiovasc. Surg. *72,* 441 (1976)
328. Stanulla, H., Dürschmied, H.: Mediastinoskopie (Indikation, Leistungsfähigkeit und morphologische Befunde bei über 2250 Untersuchungen). Z. Erkrank. Atm. Org. *144,* 12 (1976)
329. Stemmer, E.A., Calvin, J.W., Steedman, R.A., Conolly, J.E.: Parasternal mediastinal exploration to evaluate resectability of thoracic neoplasms. Ann. Thorac. Surg. *12,* 375 (1971)
330. Taube, K., Konietzko, N.: Kardiopulmonale Funktion nach Pneumonektomie präoperativ voraussagbar? Prax. Pneumol. *34,* 548 (1980)
331. Taube, K., Konietzko, N.: Prediction of postoperative cardiopulmonary function in patients undergoing pneumonectomy. Thorac. Cardiovasc. Surgeon *28,* 348 (1980)
332. Taylor, A.B.: Present position relating to cancer of the lung. Results of surgical resection. Thorax *15,* 3 (1960)
333. Thompson, D.T.: Conservative resection in surgery for bronchogenic carcinoma. J. Thorac. Cardiovasc. Surg. *53,* 159 (1967)
334. Thompson, V.C.: Present position relating to cancer of the lung. Results of resection. Thorax *15,* 5 (1960)
335. Thomsen, P.: Überlebenschancen beim ökonomisch resezierten Karzinom der Lunge anhand von 88 Fällen des Krankenhauses Großhansdorf in den Jahren 1967–1972. Prax. Pneumol. *32,* 665 (1978)
336. Töpfer, D., Riedel, L.: Erfassung von Fällen mit Bronchialkarzinom auf Grund von Beschwerden und Analyse der hierbei aufgetretenen Verschleppungszeiten. Z. Erkrank. Atm. Org. *151,* 143 (1978)
337. Trefny, J.: Erfassung des Bronchialkarzinoms in der CSSR. Z. Erkrank. Atm. Org. *150,* 250 (1978)
338. Trendelenburg, F.: Das Bronchialkarzinom als allgemeines medizinisches Problem. Prax. Pneumol. *31,* 486 (1977)
339. UICC (International Union Against Cancer): TNM-Klassifikation der malignen Tumoren. 2. Aufl. Springer, Berlin/Heidelberg/New York 1976
340. UICC (International Union Against Cancer): TNM-Klassifikation der malignen Tumoren. 3. Aufl. Springer, Berlin/Heidelberg/New York 1979
341. Ulrich, B., Ammedick, U., Berndt, V., Huth, F., Irlich, G., Konrad, R.M., Schwind, P.: Ausdehnung mediastinalen Lymphknotenbefalls beim Bronchialkarzinom in Abhängigkeit von Tumorlokalisation und Tumorart und ihre Bedeutung für die Überlebensrate. Thoraxchir. *20,* 407 (1972)
342. Ungeheuer, E., Hartel, W.: Lunge und Mediastinum. In: Therapie maligner Tumoren. Bd. II Enke, Stuttgart 1968
343. Urfer, K., Geroulanos, S., Jadoul, D., Senning, A.: Die Therapie des Pleuraempyems nach Pneumonektomie durch Thoraxfensterung bzw. kontinuierliche Spülung. Helv. chir. Acta *46,* 123 (1979)
343a. Veneskoski, T., Sovijärvi, A.R.A., Muittari, A.: Effect of lung resection on regional lung function assessed by 133-Xe radiospirometry. Lung *160,* 45 (1982)

344. Viereck, H.J.: Ergebnisse der Behandlung des Bronchialcarcinoms: operative Behandlung in Kombination mit Telekobaltbestrahlung. Pneumologie *145,* 143 (1970)
345. Vincent, R.G.: Lung Cancer – an overview. In: Perspectives in Lung Cancer. Karger, Basel 1977
346. Vincent, R.G., Takita, H., Lane, W., Gutierrez, A., Pickren, J.W.: Surgical therapy of lung cancer. J. Thorac. Cardiovasc. Surg. *71,* 581 (1976)
347. Vogel, J., Münster, Schlegel, Müller, Schnorr, Wiesner, Kandt: Präoperative Beurteilung der verbleibenden respiratorischen Funktion nach Pneumonektomie. Zeitschr. Erkrank. Atm. Org. *131,* 279 (1970)
348. Vogt-Moykopf, I., Arens, C., Zeidler, D.: Der solitäre Lungenrundherd. Eine Analyse von 636 operierten solitären Herden 1970–1976. Med. Welt *28,* 620 (1977)
349. Wannenmacher, M., Slanina, J.: Strahlentherapie des Bronchialkarzinoms. Therapiewoche *29,* 7225 (1979)
350. Wassner, U.J., Timm, J.: Zur präoperativen Ermittlung der Wahrscheinlichkeit einer pulmokardialen Insuffizienz nach Lungenresektion. Chirurg. *47,* 602 (1976)
351. Watson, L.W.: Extended surgical procedures at Memorial Hospital. In: Watson, L.W., ed.: Lung Cancer. Mosby, St. Louis 1968
352. Watson, L.W., Schottenfeld, B.: Survival and salvage rates: the patient's chance for recovery. In: Watson, L.W. (ed.): Lung cancer, a study of five thousand Memorial Hospital cases. Mosby, St. Louis 1968
353. Weiss, W., Gillick, J.S.: The metastatic spread of bronchogenic carcinoma in relation to the interval between resection and death. Chest *71,* 725 (1977)
354. Weiss, W., Boucot, K.R.: The prognosis of lung cancer as a round lesion. Data from the Philadelphia Pulmonary Neoplasm Research Project. Am. Rev. Respir. Dis. *116,* 827 (1977)
355. Weiss, W.: Operative mortality and five-year survival rates in men with bronchogenic carcinoma. Chest *66,* 483 (1974)
356. Wellons, H.A., Johnson, G., Benson, W.R., Pate, D., Wilcox, B.R., Peters, R.M.: Prognostic factors in malignant tumors of the lung. An analysis of 582 cases. Ann. Thorac. Surg. *5,* 228 (1968)
357. Wheat, M.W., Burford, T.H.: Digitalis in surgery: extension of classic indications. J. Thorac. Cardiovasc. Surg. *41,* 162 (1961)
358. Wilde, J.: Probleme der Chemotherapie beim operierten Bronchialkarzinom. Z. Erkrank. Atm. Org. *142,* 101 (1975)
359. Wilde, J.: Zur Nachsorge Bronchialkarzinomkranker. Z. Erkrank. Atm. Org. *155,* 272 (1980)
360. Wilde, J., jun., Wilde, J., sen., Ganguin, H.-G.: Röntgenologische Verschleppungszeiten beim Bronchialkarzinom. Z. Erkrank. Atm. Org. *156,* 100 (1981)
361. Wilde, J., Berzon, R., Pielesch, W., Dürschmied, H.: Die Bedeutung einer funktionellen Vorbehandlung für die Operationsfähigkeit von Bronchialkarzinomkranken. Z Erkrank. Atm. Org. *144,* 19 (1976)
362. Wilkins, E.W.: Extrathoracic manifestations of thoracic neoplasms. In: Smith, R.E. and Williams, W.G.: Surgery of the lung. The Coventry Conference, Butterworths, London 1974
362a. Wilkins, E.W., Saita, S.: Surgery for lung cancer: the Massachusetts General Hospital experience. In: Choi, N.C., Grillo, H.C., eds., Thoracic oncology, Raven Press, New York 1983
363. Wilkins, E.W., Scannell, J.G., Craver, J.G.: Four decades of experience with resections for bronchogenic carcinoma at the Massachusetts General Hospital. J. Thorac. Cardiovasg. Surg. *76,* 364 (1978)
364. Windheim v., K., Herzer, H., Schnetzer, J.: Sparsame Lungenresektionen beim peripheren Bronchialcarcinom. Pneumologie *145,* 146 (1971)
365. Wingfield, H.V.: Combined surgery and chemotherapy for carcinoma of the bronchus. Lancet *1,* 470 (1970)
366. Wulff, H.B.: Ergebnisse der chirurgischen Therapie des Bronchialcarcinoms. Langenbecks Arch. *325,* 504 (1969)

367. Wutekich, S.: Pathologie des Lungenkarzinoms. In: Denck, H., Sighart, H.: Das Bronchuskarzinom heute. Adolf Holzhausens Nachf., Wien 1980
368. Young, W.G., Perryman, R.A.: Complication of pneumonectomy. In: Cordell, A.R., Ellison, R.G., eds.: Complications of intrathoracic surgery. Little, Brown & Company, Boston 1979
369. Zeidler, D.: Die erweiterte Resektion beim Bronchialkarzinom. In: Hamelmann, H., Troidl, H.: Behandlung des Bronchialkarzinoms. Georg Thieme, Stuttgart/New York 1981
370. Zwintz, E.: Die Bedeutung der Mediastinoskopie. In: Denck, H., Sighart, H.: Das Bronchuskarzinom heute. Adolf Holzhausen Nfg., Wien 1980
371. Zwintz, E.: Anatomische Kontraindikationen zur chirurgischen Therapie des Bronchuskarzinoms. In: Denck, H., Sighart, H.: Das Bronchuskarzinom heute. Adolf Holzhausens Nachf., Wien 1980

Subject Index

GPSR Compliance
The European Union's (EU) General Product Safety Regulation (GPSR) is a set of rules that requires consumer products to be safe and our obligations to ensure this.

If you have any concerns about our products, you can contact us on

ProductSafety@springernature.com

In case Publisher is established outside the EU, the EU authorized representative is:

Springer Nature Customer Service Center GmbH
Europaplatz 3
69115 Heidelberg, Germany

www.ingramcontent.com/pod-product-compliance
Lightning Source LLC
Chambersburg PA
CBHW061214240926
51846CB00006B/1227
* 9 7 8 3 6 4 2 7 0 9 7 9 1 *